The Essential Guide TO

Asperger's Syndrome

WITHDRAWN

by Eileen Bailey
and Robert W. Montgomery, PhD

ALPHA

A member of Penguin Group (USA) Inc.

ALPHA BOOKS

Published by Penguin Group (USA) Inc.

Penguin Group (USA) Inc., 375 Hudson Street, New York, New York 10014, USA • Penguin Group (Canada), 90 Eglinton Avenue East, Suite 700, Toronto, Ontario M4P 2Y3, Canada (a division of Pearson Penguin Canada Inc.) • Penguin Books Ltd., 80 Strand, London WC2R 0RL, England • Penguin Ireland, 25 St. Stephen's Green, Dublin 2, Ireland (a division of Penguin Books Ltd.) • Penguin Group (Australia), 250 Camberwell Road, Camberwell, Victoria 3124, Australia (a division of Pearson Australia Group Pty. Ltd.) • Penguin Books India Pvt. Ltd., 11 Community Centre, Panchsheel Park, New Delhi—110 017, India • Penguin Group (NZ), 67 Apollo Drive, Rosedale, North Shore, Auckland 1311, New Zealand (a division of Pearson New Zealand Ltd.) • Penguin Books (South Africa) (Pty.) Ltd., 24 Sturdee Avenue, Rosebank, Johannesburg 2196, South Africa

Penguin Books Ltd., Registered Offices: 80 Strand, London WC2R 0RL, England

International Standard Book Number: 978-1-61564-165-9
Library of Congress Catalog Card Number: 2011943392

14   13   12   8   7   6   5   4   3   2

Interpretation of the printing code: The rightmost number of the first series of numbers is the year of the book's printing; the rightmost number of the second series of numbers is the number of the book's printing. For example, a printing code of 12-1 shows that the first printing occurred in 2012.

Printed in the United States of America

Note: This publication contains the opinions and ideas of its authors. It is intended to provide helpful and informative material on the subject matter covered. It is sold with the understanding that the authors and publisher are not engaged in rendering professional services in the book. If the reader requires personal assistance or advice, a competent professional should be consulted.

The authors and publisher specifically disclaim any responsibility for any liability, loss, or risk, personal or otherwise, which is incurred as a consequence, directly or indirectly, of the use and application of any of the contents of this book.

Most Alpha books are available at special quantity discounts for bulk purchases for sales promotions, premiums, fund-raising, or educational use. Special books, or book excerpts, can also be created to fit specific needs.

For details, write: Special Markets, Alpha Books, 375 Hudson Street, New York, NY 10014.

Publisher: *Marie Butler-Knight*
Associate Publisher: *Mike Sanders*
Executive Managing Editor: *Billy Fields*
Senior Acquisitions Editor: *Brook Farling*
Development Editor: *Mark Reddin*
Senior Production Editor: *Kayla Dugger*
Copy Editor: *Kelly D. Henthorne*

Cover Designer: *Rebecca Batchelor*
Book Designers: *Rebecca Batchelor, William Thomas*
Indexer: *Celia McCoy*
Layout: *Brian Massey*
Proofreader: *John Etchison*

Dedications

Eileen Bailey:

Dedicated to my son, Soloman, the self-diagnosed Aspie in my life who continually shows me the wonder and positive side of Asperger's syndrome.

Robert Montgomery:

To my children, Rob and Kate, for helping me see through your eyes.

Contents

Appendixes

Introduction

When parents first receive a diagnosis of Asperger's syndrome (AS), they usually have more questions than answers. Is it autism? Is it high-functioning autism? Is it mild autism? What does it mean? Will our child grow out of it? Will he be able to go to college? Will he be able to work? Can he feel love?

AS is a relatively new diagnosis. Although first described by Hans Asperger in 1944, it did not gain much attention until 1981 when Lorna Wing, a researcher who had a daughter with autism, challenged the accepted definition of autism. In 1994, the term Asperger's syndrome was added as an official diagnosis, separate from autism, and acceptance of the diagnosis has grown since then, although it is still commonly misunderstood.

AS is a pervasive developmental disorder characterized by difficulty with socialization and communication, repetitive actions, and an intense focus on a specific topic. A number of secondary symptoms are common in children with AS, such as sensory sensitivities and clumsiness. No single treatment is available for AS, rather a child's individual symptoms are considered in a customized treatment plan that may include physical therapy, occupational therapy, speech therapy, and social skills training.

If your child has recently been diagnosed with AS, or even if you don't have an official diagnosis but think your child may have AS, this book can answer many of your questions. If you have been dealing with a diagnosis for several years, this book offers suggestions, tips, and a deeper understanding of your child's behaviors.

Friends and relatives may also find this book helpful in better understanding some of your child's behaviors. For those who interact with your child on a regular basis, this book can provide a resource for not only understanding but how their actions can help to teach your child social skills. It is our hope that we have provided you with answers to your questions; new information, tips, and suggestions on how to deal with specific behaviors; and a new way of looking at how your child sees the world.

Throughout this book we have used the term "him" to describe a child with AS. This is not meant to imply that girls do not have AS; it has been used for simplicity of writing. We understand that girls can and do have AS and included a chapter that specifically addresses issues faced by girls with AS.

How to Use This Book

Let's start with what isn't in this book. You won't find a lot of medical jargon or hard-to-understand language. We've written it so that you, the parents, can find the information you need without wading through medical terminology. In cases where this type of language is necessary, we've provided you with an explanation. At the end of the book is a glossary of commonly used terminology within the Aspie world for your reference. We have also provided a list of resources, with organizations, websites, and books to help you find additional information.

This book is divided into six different parts to make it easier to find the information you need:

Part 1, Overview of Asperger's Syndrome, covers much of the basic information. It explains what AS is and how it differs from autism. It covers how the proposed changes to the diagnostic criteria can impact medical care for your child. We explain the early warning signs and some of the common secondary symptoms and address specific issues related to girls with AS. We also discuss other conditions commonly associated with AS. Finally, we talk about what treatments are available and how you go about creating a treatment team to best help your child.

Part 2, Behaviors, covers thought processes and behaviors. We explain the differences and similarities between tantrums and meltdowns and offer ideas on how to manage meltdowns, both in your home and in public. We discuss repetitive behaviors, giving insight into how these behaviors and rituals provide a sense of security to your child. We talk about the literal and logical thought processes of individuals with AS and give ideas on how to use this to better communicate with your child. We discuss why many children with AS are perfectionists. Finally, we address how these behaviors change during the different stages of your child's development, from infancy to young adulthood.

Part 3, Managing Obsessions, covers one of the hallmark characteristics of AS, special interests or passions. We provide explanations on how special interests benefit your child and help create a sense of security. We discuss the differences between quickly changing passions and those that last through a lifetime and what parents can do when special interests are inappropriate. We offer ways parents can use special interests to help in teaching children social, academic, and communication skills. We discuss how special interests, like behaviors, change over time, from the early years when your child might be fixated on a part of a toy to the young adult years, when passions can lead to employment.

Part 4, Social Skills, covers the most difficult area for Aspies, social interactions. We first discuss what social competence means and where children with AS most often have problems. In each subsequent chapter, we talk about a specific age group and how social skills deficits impact their relationships. We begin with young children, explaining the differences between parallel play and cooperative play and discuss weaknesses in reciprocal play at this stage. We provide insight into some of the difficulties for elementary age children, such as recognizing personal space, aggression, and knowing when to be totally honest and when to use tact. We explore some of the problems in the preteen and teen years, both in friendship and dating, and offer parents suggestions on how to help their child through this difficult time in their life. We address the issue of bullying, discussing why Aspies are often targeted by bullies, how parents can recognize signs that their child is being bullied, and strategies for parents. Finally, we talk about young adults and discuss social skills both in the college and work environments as well as helping your young adult learn to live independently.

Part 5, Educational Considerations, covers different aspects of working within the educational system to help your child throughout his school years. We discuss Early Intervention (EI) programs as well as different ways your child can receive special services at school. We discuss the process of requesting services and working with education professionals as well as how you can work as your child's advocate. We provide examples of special services that have worked for other children with AS, and finally we offer ways to help your child develop self-help skills to improve academic and social skills.

Part 6, You and Your Family, covers how AS impacts family life. We discuss how you might react when first given a diagnosis of AS and provide help on finding ways to relieve some of the stress of living with a child with special needs. We talk about the importance of focusing on your relationship with your spouse. We explain the importance of providing structure in your home but warn about the dangers of creating a too structured environment. We provide insight on how AS impacts siblings and give ideas for helping them cope with having a sibling with AS. Finally, we address the challenges of attending events with your Aspie and how to make these outings successful. We offer ideas on talking to friends and relatives about your child's diagnosis and how to respond to negative comments.

Essential Extras

Throughout the book, you'll see additional pieces of information in sidebars. Here's what to look for:

Definition	These sidebars offer definitions of words or phrases that may be unfamiliar to you.

Aspie Advice	Look here for general AS-related tips and guidance for you and your Aspie loved one.

The Doctor's Take	These are warnings and other special considerations relevant to the topic offered by Dr. Montgomery.

You'll also see a fourth, name-changing sidebar that presents anecdotes, interesting facts, case histories, or other extended background information you should know.

Acknowledgments

Eileen Bailey: Many thanks to my husband, George, who, as always, gave me love, support, and encouragement as I wrote this book. I also must thank my son, Soloman, who never ceases to show me, as a self-diagnosed Aspie, the wonder and positive side of Asperger's syndrome. And many thanks to my daughter Evelyn, who always brings a smile to my face. My deepest appreciation to my neighbors, Paul and Sandy Raegler, who generously shared stories, explanations, and a wonderful sense of humor about raising twins with autism. Thank you to all the parents who offered their insights about raising, living with, and loving children with AS. With great appreciation to Paula Gardner, PhD, who helped me understand how AS impacts a child at school and who provided tips for parents; and Laura Stephens, PhD, who shared her knowledge on early warning signs of AS. And last but not least, many thanks to my co-author, Robert, who shared his wealth of knowledge of AS to help make sure this book is accurate and full of practical tips and suggestions for parents raising a child with AS.

Robert Montgomery: My sincere appreciation goes to all the children, adolescents, and adults with Asperger's whom I have had the pleasure of working with over the years—those interactions were the real education for me. My thanks also to Eileen for all her encouragement and understanding through this process. My appreciation to my two mentors, Ted Ayllon and Michael Milan, for teaching me many things, not least among them that the more you know, the more you can help others. And to my father, who only had one question for me and it taught me a lot: "Did you do your best son?" Finally, to my family for making it all worth it.

Both Eileen and Robert would like to thank our agent, Marilyn Allen, and the editors, Brook Farling, Mark Reddin, and Kayla Dugger, who all worked hard to make this book a reality.

Trademarks

All terms mentioned in this book that are known to be or are suspected of being trademarks or service marks have been appropriately capitalized. Alpha Books and Penguin Group (USA) Inc. cannot attest to the accuracy of this information. Use of a term in this book should not be regarded as affecting the validity of any trademark or service mark.

Part 1

Overview of Asperger's Syndrome

Whether your child was recently diagnosed with Asperger's syndrome (AS) or was diagnosed years ago, as a parent, you probably have more questions than answers. You might wonder how AS differs from autism or what causes AS. Part 1 answers many of these questions.

Currently, the average age of diagnosis in the United States is 11 to 12 years old. That means many parents have spent years living with symptoms they didn't understand, meltdowns, their child's lack of friends or inability to make friends, sensory sensitivities, and communication problems. They may have had a string of other diagnoses, such as Attention Deficit Hyperactivity Disorder (ADHD) or obsessive compulsive disorder (OCD). We explain which disorders are commonly confused with AS and which are often seen alongside AS.

The majority of children diagnosed with AS are boys, although it isn't yet understood whether it is more prevalent in boys or if the symptoms of AS show up differently in girls and are ignored. We discuss what AS looks like in girls and some of the special issues that go along with the diagnosis, especially as girls reach puberty and begin entering into relationships.

chapter 1

Understanding Asperger's Syndrome

Checklist of Asperger's syndrome behaviors

Differences between Asperger's syndrome and autism

How changes in the diagnostic criteria affect your child

How Asperger's syndrome is diagnosed

Asperger's syndrome was first researched more than 60 years ago by Hans Asperger. He published the first definition of Asperger's syndrome in 1944 and opened a school for children with what are today considered autistic symptoms. His work went largely unnoticed until the 1990s, when Lorna Wing, one of the founders of the National Autistic Society, researched autism and challenged the medical community's definition of autism. She was the first person to use the phrase "Asperger's syndrome," and her findings drew attention to Hans Asperger's research. Today this condition is well accepted yet still largely misunderstood and—according to some experts—underdiagnosed, especially in girls.

What Is Asperger's Syndrome?

Asperger's syndrome (AS) is a developmental disorder characterized by unusual and intense preoccupation with a subject, impaired social and communication skills, and repetitive behaviors. It is an *autism spectrum disorder,* and it is estimated that 2 out of every 10,000 children have AS. Boys are currently diagnosed four times more often than girls.

Definition

Autism spectrum disorders are a group of developmental disorders also known as pervasive developmental disorders (PDD). Besides AS, this group includes autistic disorder, pervasive development disorder—not otherwise specified, Rett syndrome, and childhood disintegrative disorder.

Just as each child is unique, the symptoms of AS appear differently in each one. Because it is considered a spectrum disorder, your child may show only mild symptoms, and another child may show more severe symptoms. Some children may show a number of AS traits, others only a few. This can make it confusing for you as a parent because you may see some traits in your child that another child with AS doesn't have. The following is a checklist of many of the common AS traits. As you read through the list, pay particular attention to those traits that resonate with your recent feelings and check all that you feel may apply. This is a great tool to bring along to your initial doctor's appointment to help explain some of the behaviors you are seeing in your child.

Social and Communication Skills

- ❏ May interact with adults more than with other children
- ❏ Does not "pretend" or engage in imaginative play
- ❏ Avoids eye contact with adults and other children
- ❏ Seems to not listen or ignores people when they speak
- ❏ Talks a lot about a particular interest
- ❏ Doesn't "get" sarcasm or jokes
- ❏ Speaks in monotone or sing-song voice
- ❏ Has difficulty making friends even though there is a desire to make friends

❐ Doesn't understand rules of play commonly understood by other children

❐ Shows an apparent lack of empathy

❐ Can't read emotions on other people's faces

❐ Has difficulty understanding nonverbal communication

The Doctor's Take

People with auditory, or hearing, sensitivities sometimes hear and are disturbed by sounds other people don't hear or pay attention to—for example, the buzz from fluorescent lighting.

Sensory Sensitivities

❐ Highly sensitive to sound; may cover ears or cry around loud noises

❐ Sensitive to touch; refuses to wear certain fabrics or needs all tags removed from clothing

❐ Sensitive to different textures of food; only eats certain food

❐ Doesn't like having food, finger paint, or other substances on hands

❐ Prefers to not get wet—doesn't like baths, showers, or swimming

Cognitive Skills

❐ Literal, or linear, thinking process

❐ Reads at a young age

❐ Memorizes books if they match interests

❐ Has an extensive vocabulary

❐ Intense interest in a particular subject; seems to be obsessed with this interest

❐ Good at remembering facts, dates, and figures even when the concept behind the information isn't understood

❐ Likes routines and rituals; tense and irritable if schedule is changed

Motor Skills

    ❏ Lack of coordination; clumsy

    ❏ Difficulty learning to ride a bike, scooter, or skates

    ❏ Doesn't do well in sports

    ❏ Problems learning to tie shoes

    ❏ Illegible or messy handwriting

    ❏ Finds it hard to use utensils

    ❏ Delay in fine motor skills

If you have checked some of the previously listed traits and characteristics, it does not mean your child has AS, but you may want to speak with your family doctor or pediatrician and work together to decide whether further evaluation is necessary.

Asperger's Syndrome vs. Autism

AS is one disorder in the autistic spectrum disorders. The lines between autism and AS are sometimes blurry because symptoms overlap—for example, communication and social problems are apparent in both. The following sections explain the similarities and differences between autism and AS.

Speech

Children with AS do not generally have speech delays. The diagnostic criteria in the *Diagnostic and Statistical Manual, Fourth Edition,* states there are "no significant language delays" in children with AS; even so, language abilities and development do vary in children with AS. Some children are very verbal, using an extensive, formal vocabulary at a young age but have trouble communicating their needs and wants. For example, your child can name his colors or memorize a favorite book but can't tell you what he wants to eat. Other concerns with speech development are unusual speech patterns and talking in a monotone or sing-song manner. Your child might also have difficulty with pragmatics, understanding abstract and social uses of language.

> **Definition**
>
> The ***Diagnostic and Statistical Manual*** **(DSM)** is published by the American Psychiatric Association and provides diagnostic criteria for all mental illnesses. It is used to classify, describe, and diagnose mental disorders. There have been five updates since it was first published in the 1950s, and a sixth update is expected in 2013.

Generally more significant language problems occur in autism than in AS. A child with autism might start speaking late; some never speak. Most children with autism do eventually use some type of spoken language or learn to communicate through sign language or pictures. Some even begin talking around age 1 but lose the ability to speak by around 2 years of age. This can be a gradual process, or your child may suddenly stop speaking. If this happens, you should immediately talk with your doctor.

Cognitive Skills

As with speech delays, delays in cognitive skills normally do not occur in children with AS but might in children with autism. "Cognitive skills" refers to our ability to learn and use our thoughts, experiences, and senses to obtain and understand information. A study completed by the University of Illinois–Chicago found that between 40 percent and 75 percent of individuals with autism had cognitive impairment, with IQ scores less than 70. Some specific areas children with autism have difficulties are:

Visuospatial coherence. The ability to see an object as separate parts and then put those parts together such as buttoning a shirt, putting together a puzzle, and making a bed.

False-belief understanding. The ability to infer what other people believe and think and then predict behavior. For example, suppose your child moves a toy while you are out of the room. He will understand you don't know where the toy is, but a child with underdeveloped false-belief understanding assumes you know where the toy is because he knows where it is. This usually occurs after 2 years of age.

High-Functioning Autism vs. Asperger's Syndrome

misc.   You may hear the term "high-functioning autism" to describe someone with AS. This term is generally used to describe someone who meets the definition of autism but later developed speech. Those diagnosed with AS usually do not have any speech delays.

Executive functioning. Using cognitive abilities to carry out daily tasks such as planning, organization, keeping track of time, multitasking, recalling past events and relating them to the current situation, changing plans when needed, and interacting with a group of people.

Social Skills and Communication

Children with AS and those with autism have problems with social skills and communication. Those with AS tend to be more interested in developing social bonds than those with autism but still need to be taught basic social skills, such as looking someone in the eye, recognizing facial expressions, and participating in a conversation. Some children with AS are considered "odd" or socially inept, and a diagnosis of AS is overlooked because symptoms are usually milder than those with autism.

The Changing Face of Asperger's Syndrome

As explained earlier in this chapter, the DSM contains the diagnostic criteria for all mental disorders and illnesses. In 1994, AS was listed as a separate disorder; prior to that, it was diagnosed as an autism spectrum disorder. A new edition of the DSM is due out in 2013, and proposed changes will eliminate the separate diagnosis of AS and put it back under autism. This proposed change is controversial, and proponents are on both sides of the debate. However, many people with AS see this change as a mistake.

Current Description of AS

The current description of AS includes symptoms in two major categories: (1) social interactions; (2) repetitive behaviors, interests, and activities.

Symptoms must be severe enough to cause significant impairment, which means the level of symptoms interferes with your child's ability to complete or participate in normal daily activities compared to other children of the same age.

Social interaction impairment must include at least two of the following:

- Problems understanding nonverbal behaviors
- The absence of relationships with other children
- Not sharing happiness, enjoyment, interests, or achievements with others
- Difficulty with social or emotional interactions

Children with AS also exhibit repetitive behaviors, interests, and activities, including at least one of the following:

- Intense preoccupation with one or more interests
- Needing strict routines or rituals
- Repetitive movements, such as hand flapping
- Strong interest in parts of objects

Besides listing specific symptoms, the current DSM definition of AS states that delays in language or cognitive skills are not generally seen in children with AS. Further, it explains that a child cannot meet the criteria for a different pervasive development disorder or schizophrenia.

Changes That Could Affect Medical Care

According to proponents of the elimination of AS from the DSM, the major difference between AS and autism is the lack of a language delay. Other differences, such as social skills, can be explained as different levels, or ranges, of the same symptoms. AS is sometimes referred to as *high-functioning autism* to reflect the similarities. In some areas of the country, children with AS have a harder time receiving services than those diagnosed with autism. If the proposed change in the DSM takes place, children with pervasive developmental disorder, AS, and Rett syndrome would all be diagnosed with autism spectrum disorder. Proponents of the change believe it will make access to services easier for all children on the autism spectrum.

As we explain in Chapter 4, a number of common co-existing and related medical conditions occur with AS, such as anxiety, attention problems, sleep problems, and sensory issues. These conditions are frequently seen in children with autism as well. The plans for the new edition of the DSM include information about these other conditions, giving medical professionals more complete information. Proponents of the change believe this will result in your child receiving better overall medical care, with doctors taking all related conditions into account and treating the entire patient rather than treating a single disorder.

Creating one diagnosis ends the confusion created by diagnoses in flux throughout a person's life. For example, your child may meet the criteria for pervasive development disorder at one point, AS at another point, and autism at another. Using an umbrella diagnosis of "autism spectrum disorders" would eliminate the need to continually change the diagnosis or classification if your child's symptoms change.

What Is an Aspie?

MISC.

The term "Aspie" was coined by Liane Holliday Willey in 1999 and is meant to be used as a shortened, easier way to say, "a person with Asperger's syndrome." It is widely accepted and used by parents of children with AS and many adults with AS.

Those against the proposed changes, however, argue that changing the diagnosis classification is a step backward. The public (and many people who have been diagnosed with AS) view people with AS as more capable and less disabled. They believe having to list a diagnosis of autism would cause school personnel, potential employers, and even friends and relatives to look at them differently. Another concern is that because autism is characterized by speech delays, doctors will be less likely to diagnose autism if these children do not have language delays, resulting in children missing out on receiving the help and services they need.

Causes of AS

No one yet knows the exact causes of AS. The National Institutes of Health (NIH) indicates that recent research shows abnormalities in the brain. These studies show both structural and functional differences in the brains of those with AS when compared to the brains of those without AS. Some indications suggest that AS runs in families. Although additional family members may not fit the exact diagnostic criteria for AS, a higher number of family members have some of the same behaviors, even if to a lesser degree.

The Doctor's Take	It is very common for parents to want to know the cause for their child having AS, but there is currently no way to know. If someone tells you that they can definitely tell you why, it's time to seek help elsewhere.

A few unproven theories exist about the possible cause of AS:

- Some people believe vaccines that contain mercury can lead to autism or AS. Mercury poisoning has similar symptoms as those found in autism or AS, and many parents indicate their child lost speech abilities shortly after receiving the measles, mumps, and rubella vaccine (MMR). Recent investigations around the world have failed to support this as a cause for increases in autism spectrum disorders (ASD).

- Allergies to certain foods are also named by some as a possible cause of AS. In particular, gluten and casein have been named as culprits. While a few parents saw noticeable improvements in their child's behaviors when foods containing gluten or casein were removed from their diets, many others saw no change at all.

These are simply theories about what may cause Asperger's, and there is no definitive answer. It was previously thought that AS was caused by emotional deprivation. Today, many people may mistakenly see AS behaviors as rudeness and assume these are the result of poor parenting skills. Even though the exact causes are unknown, we now know that poor parenting does not cause AS.

Looking for Answers

AS is diagnosed most often based on the lack of social skills, which makes it highly unlikely that an AS diagnosis is accurate prior to Kindergarten age. You may have noticed differences in your child from a young age, such as his lack of pretend play or that he continued to play alongside other children rather than with them. As with many parents, you may have viewed this as immaturity, assuming your child would develop social skills after he entered school. As your child matures and still doesn't seem to be able to make friends, has frequent meltdowns, or is having problems in school, you, as parents, seek help from your pediatrician or family doctor. Normally, your doctor does not complete an assessment for AS but refers you to a pediatric psychologist or psychiatrist with expertise in AS for an evaluation. Your child's school may request a private evaluation, but it is also important to know that the school may be required under various state and federal regulations (e.g., IDEA 2004, PL 94–142, etc.) to evaluate your child for possible supports and accommodations.

What's Involved in an Evaluation?

Your child's evaluation begins with questions about why you believe your child has AS. You can use the checklist in the beginning of this chapter as a starting point, explaining what symptoms you notice in your child and offering some examples of your child's behaviors. Depending on your child's age, the doctor might also ask him questions directly.

> **The Doctor's Take**
>
> An evaluation for AS could upset your child's routine. To help your child, talk about the upcoming appointment, letting your child know this doctor will only ask questions (no shots). You might also want to show him where the office is on a map or take a dry run to the office to ease his fears. Let him know the day and time of the appointment, what time you are leaving, and when you expect to be home. For many children with Asperger's, the more information you share, the easier it is.

You will probably be asked to complete a rating scale. A number of different rating scales help a doctor evaluate your child's symptoms and behaviors. The following are examples of questions on a rating scale:

- Does the child lack awareness of how to play with other children? For example, does the child seem unaware of unwritten rules of social play?

- Does the child lack social imaginative play? For example, does the child not seem to understand pretend play?

When completing a rating scale, you are asked to indicate whether this behavior is seen rarely, frequently, or somewhere in between. In addition to these types of questions, you are asked to mark off whether your child shows certain other traits, such as anxiety in noisy places; an extreme dislike or sensitivity to ordinary sounds, such as an appliance running or fluorescent lights; or behaviors such as flapping his hands. On such scales, you are also asked about your child's interests. Take your time, don't over-analyze, and if you have a question, ask the professional conducting the evaluation. They want accurate and clear information, and your questions should help them to understand your child better.

> **Aspie Advice**
>
> The more information you bring to your initial consultation, the better your doctor can complete an evaluation. If your child had previous psychological, neurological, or other medical evaluations—including illnesses and surgeries—bring a copy of the reports. If your child is currently receiving special education services, bring along a copy of the current Individualized Educational Plan (IEP), the eligibility report, and all evaluation reports including information on behavior and academic progress.

Your doctor will also ask you about your child's development. He wants to know when your child spoke his first word, when several words were put together to form sentences, when he rolled over, and when he walked. Specific psychological tests, such as IQ and language tests, are frequently completed as part of the evaluation. Some additional ways your doctor evaluates your child include:

- Talking with your child to find out whether he can talk about a variety of subjects or if there is a narrow focus during conversations

- Observing to see whether your child makes eye contact

- Asking your child how a person in a picture is feeling based on facial expression

- Having your child catch and throw a ball or draw a picture to assess motor coordination

- Listening to your child's speech patterns and inflections while speaking

If your child has been seen by other therapists, such as speech or occupational therapists, your doctor should request those reports. It is a good idea to take all records related to your child from any evaluations with you to the diagnostic appointment. This can save time and help better inform the doctor from the start. He might give you a questionnaire for your child's teacher to complete. Your doctor gathers all of the information together and reviews it. It usually takes several weeks to receive a written report from the doctor.

Confusion with Other Disorders and Conditions

A number of disorders and conditions have symptoms that overlap with AS. Some of the behaviors, such as difficulty in social situations, look similar to a withdrawal in social settings caused by other conditions. It is important for your doctor to look for other possible reasons before determining your child has AS. Some of the common conditions sometimes confused with AS are:

- Language or other learning disabilities

- Nonverbal learning disorder (NVLD)

- Attention Deficit Hyperactivity Disorder (ADHD)

- Anxiety

- Giftedness

The Doctor's Take

Diagnosing AS is sometimes difficult because, in addition to sharing symptoms with other conditions and disorders, it is possible to have more than one condition. For example, your child can have both AS and ADHD. It is important to find a medical professional with expertise in AS who understands the differences—for example, a level of focus is expected in children with AS that is not expected in children with ADHD.

It is possible a child is extremely shy or introverted. A complete and thorough evaluation by a qualified, experienced medical professional can rule out other possible causes of your child's symptoms, provide an accurate diagnosis, and set up a plan of action.

Essential Takeaways

- AS is characterized by impaired social skills, intense preoccupation with a subject, and repetitive behaviors.

- Symptoms of autism and AS can overlap, but there are also distinct differences, such as in language and cognition.

- The criteria for diagnosing AS may change within the next few years, impacting your child's medical treatment.

- A psychologist or psychiatrist completes a thorough evaluation of social skills, interests, abilities, and behaviors to determine whether a child has AS.

chapter 2

Symptoms

Early behaviors that can signal AS

Why children with AS have a hard time making friends

AS and rigid thinking

Problems in language development

How hypersensitivities affect a child with AS

Asperger's syndrome (AS) is one of the "invisible dis-abilities." You can't see it or feel it. No blood test or other high-tech scan can let you know your child has AS. When a person meets your child, she won't say, "Oh, I see he has Asperger's syndrome." But from a young age your child exhibits signs, both clear and sub-tle, and as he grows, symptoms typically become more noticeable.

Early Warning Signs

AS is not normally diagnosed before the age of 4 and often is not diagnosed until after a child begins school, when the lack of social interactions becomes apparent. Many parents, however, are concerned about certain behaviors, even before their child's first or second birthday. Sometimes, these signs go unnoticed; maybe because parents have a hard time admitting some-thing is wrong or maybe because parents accept the peculiar behaviors as normal. This is especially true for first-time parents who have no frame of reference for behaviors in infants and young children. For these parents, abnormal behaviors appear to be quirks of personality.

Early identification of AS has definite advantages. Early Intervention (EI) programs greatly improve your child's ability to learn appropriate behaviors and social skills. Research has shown these types of skills are best learned when taught at an early age, when your child is still developing. Research also tells us that social skills and the ability to positively interact with others are much better predictors of success than intelligence and mastery of skills and information. We also now understand that the earlier these skills are learned, the easier the child will adapt to a variety of social situations throughout their life span.

Much of the research on early warning signs is specific to autism but the amount of information on the early development of Aspies is growing. Dr. Laura Stephens, the Director of Clinical Services at Education Spectrum, has worked with children with AS for over 20 years and specializes in the early diagnosis of AS.

The Doctor's Take

Diagnosing AS in young children is very controversial because it is difficult to identify social deficits, a central component of an AS diagnosis, in children under the age of 6 or 7.

Dr. Stephens suggests that some key characteristics in young children can be as follows:

- May be fussy or colicky as infants; normal comforting strategies may not work but may be comforted by the hum of a fan

- May be more interested in objects than people

- May be agitated around strangers

- May have unusual first words, such as "light" or "shoe"

- Confusion of pronouns, such as saying "You are hungry" rather than "I am hungry"

- May have difficulty with understanding figures of speech, such as "I am running to the store" (thinking you are literally going to run)

- Sees each object with singular purpose and doesn't understand toys can be played with in multiple ways

- May not point to objects

- May not wave "hi" or "bye"

- Doesn't interact with other children

- Does not engage in pretend play

- Becomes irritable and cranky when situations change, even small changes such as using a different blanket or rearranging furniture

- May want the same food every day or may only eat one or two different foods

- May have sensory issues, such as not liking loud noises, bright lights, or tags in clothing

- May develop an intense interest in a topic as toddlers

- May play with only certain toys, such as blue toys, or may be more interested in taking toys apart than playing with them

Knowing such early indicators can help you decide whether your child should see a doctor. Because of the difficulty in diagnosing young children, seek out a doctor who specializes in children with AS.

Four Major Symptoms of AS

In Chapter 1, we talked about some of the common traits of Aspies as well as the diagnostic criteria. In this chapter, we discuss the main symptoms of AS and how each manifests in children. In later chapters we look at each of these symptoms and talk about specific behaviors and how parents can cope with and manage different behaviors at different ages.

Aspie Advice

Your child needs to be taught the basics of social interaction. This includes greeting people, starting a conversation, taking turns during a conversation, and ending a conversation. One way of teaching conversation skills is to role-play. Remember, children with AS often find it easier interacting with adults but don't forget to practice with peers as well!

Social Deficiencies

Joshua watched as the other boys played together, desperately wanting to join in. He felt his loneliness intensely but was afraid and didn't know what to say. Finally, he went over to the group of boys, held up the model truck in his hand, and said, "The Ford F150 gets 22 miles per gallon." The boys looked at him and asked his name. He didn't answer the question; instead he recited more facts about pick-up trucks. The group of boys slowly moved away, finding other things to do. Joshua was dejected. No matter how much he wanted friends, he never seemed to say the right thing.

Many Aspies very much want to make friends but lack the social skills. Most also appear to prefer solitary play and often resist someone entering their "space," but many deeply feel the pain of isolation. Aspies may have an extensive vocabulary but don't understand the nuances of other people's speech. For example, simple statements such as "That's cool" bring visions of cool temperatures, and the phrase meaning that something is desirable eludes Aspies.

As with Joshua, conversations are usually one-sided and lack the give and take of effective communication. One topic, or passion, dominates the conversation. In Joshua's case it was pick-up trucks, but in Chapter 8 we explain that special interests are varied from child to child and can be on any topic, some of no interest to other children, such as washing machines or how air conditioners work. Some Aspies repetitively state the same question or statement. Joshua, instead of reciting different facts about trucks, might have repeated the fact about gas mileage. Because an Aspie is so genuinely interested in a topic, he lacks the realization that other people do not find it fascinating.

Children without AS use different speech inflections. Most children's voices become shriller when excited; their speech becomes faster when passionate; they talk more slowly when sad. Aspies may talk in monotones or in a sing-song voice. Their faces are usually expressionless, and Aspies don't often use other nonverbal signals to show feelings.

Other children don't know or understand this limited communication and shy away from spending time with or talking to the child with AS. Aspies may prefer to spend time with one or two other people, with whom they feel comfortable. Many times Aspies are more at ease with adults or older children rather than peers.

Rigid Thinking

Andrea was spending the day at her cousin Laura's house. Andrea and Laura were both 4 years old. Aunt Marie was busy cleaning the house while the girls sat quietly drawing. When Aunt Marie was done sweeping the kitchen, she propped the broom against the wall and moved on to dusting the living room. Laura jumped up, grabbed the broom, and ran around the house "riding" the broom, pretending she was riding a horse. Andrea stared, completely confused. Why was Laura jumping around and yelling while holding a broom between her legs? A broom is for sweeping floors.

MISC.

Rigid Thinking

Rigid thinking shows up in many aspects of life, not just in social situations. Your child may want to do homework in a certain order or certain way and is not open to new ideas. He may need to sit in the same chair to watch television or get dressed in a certain way. Any changes in an established routine can throw him off balance.

Andrea, like most Aspies, didn't understand pretend play. Her rigid, literal thinking allowed her to see objects only in one way. When Andrea played with blocks at home, she was adept at re-creating buildings her mother made but lacked the imagination to create new building designs. When interacting with other children, Andrea, and other children with AS, might seem bossy because they want to play only certain games and play according to established rules. These Aspies aren't trying to be bossy; this is the way they feel safe and secure and is the only way they understand how to play. Aspies don't comprehend that other people have different opinions and assume everyone else sees the world exactly as they do—linear and organized.

Obsessions

Obsessions, as we discuss in Chapter 8, are also known as special interests; a more positive term for them is "passions." The term obsession denotes something negative and is often rejected by Aspies and their families while the term "passion" conveys a more positive image. Sometimes special interests lead to employment. For example, an intense interest in computers can build skills as a repair technician or software developer. These interests, however, are sometimes frustrating for parents and family members because they dominate conversations and social outings.

> **Definition**
>
> An **obsession** is a fixation on an idea, object, or person. Thoughts and ideas about the obsession intrude in a person's thoughts and interfere with normal functioning for the person. While obsessions, such as those in obsessive compulsive disorder (OCD), are unwanted and intrusive, obsessions in children with AS are a passionate interest.

These interests do offer benefits, giving your child a way to relax, a sense of order in his life, and a way to increase self-esteem. Some passions last only a few weeks, ending as suddenly as they began, while others last throughout your child's life. Parents and teachers can incorporate special interests into lessons for reading, math, and other subjects as well as use them to help teach social skills.

Because many children with AS spend as much time as possible researching, talking about, or interacting with an interest, you sometimes need to limit access. Some parents use interests as a motivator, allowing access when homework or chores have been completed.

Differences in Language Development

Aspies do not usually have delays in language development. They say their first word around 12 months old and are able to string words together into phrases and sentences around the same age as children without AS (usually around 2 years of age). They can develop extensive vocabularies, which sometimes contain technical terms related to their passions. Vocabulary consists mainly of verbs and nouns; adjectives and adverbs are used infrequently. Aspies are sometimes referred to as "little professors" because of an ability to talk about a specific topic at length and the monotone delivery of the information. Aspies frequently use speech to convey information about a special interest but typically do not convey feelings, emotions, or thoughts.

A Passion for Electrical Outlets

Misc.

Billy, beginning around age 5, would approach adults and tell them, in great detail, about the different types of electrical outlets. He could name many companies that made the outlets, the different types, and that they are different in other countries. Many adults were fascinated that this little boy was interested in outlets and knew so much about them. However, whenever Billy was at someone else's house, instead of interacting with the other children, he would wander around looking at each outlet.

Following are some areas where language development differs from children without AS:

Uses scripts when talking. Scripts can be from a television show, video game, or movie or can be made up to fit certain situations. Scripts are, at times, unnoticeable, and at other times sound like nonsense talk.

Talks incessantly about special interest. Once your child begins talking about his passion, it is as if he can't stop.

Sounds robotic. Aspies have impairment in *prosody* and do not vary the rhythm of speech or will speak too softly or too loudly. Aspies may use voices from cartoons, not understanding this is not appropriate in conversation.

Prosody with regard to spoken language refers to intonation and stress patterns. This includes the pitch, rhythm, and melody of speech.

Definition

Difficulty processing auditory information. Sometimes a delay occurs in responding to another person because spoken information needs to be processed and analyzed. Aspies have a hard time differentiating relevant and nonrelevant information in conversations. This is actually an issue of comprehension, but many parents have their child evaluated by an audiologist to make sure the child is not having difficulty hearing.

Secondary Symptoms of AS

While motor skills deficiencies and sensory sensitivities are not listed among the main symptoms of AS, many Aspies have problems in the following areas.

Motor Skills

Clumsy, physically awkward, uncoordinated—all these words have been used often to describe Aspies. Many children with AS are gifted in other areas, such as art, music, or computers. It is rare to find a gifted athlete who has AS, although they do exist. They are often developmentally late at activities requiring gross and fine motor skills, such as holding a pencil, tying shoes, catching a ball, riding a bike, or using the monkey bars at the playground.

> **Aspie Advice**
>
> To help your child improve fine motor skills, roll play dough into small pea-size balls using only fingertips or cut play dough with plastic utensils. Each requires fine motor control, is very forgiving if mistakes are made, and gives your child good tactile feedback.

Deficits in motor skills frequently cause problems at school, causing frustration for Aspies because they are not able to do things their classmates do. Aspies may be afraid to try new things or have illegible handwriting. Difficulties holding a pencil interfere with completing school assignments. Being clumsy and uncoordinated causes embarrassment in gym class or feelings of inferiority when attempting different sports or physical activities, even playing on the playground.

Research into AS and physical movement is ongoing, and some researchers believe understanding how motor skills are affected by AS can lead to earlier diagnosis in the future. For example, a study completed at the University of Florida by Osnat and Philip Teitelbaum reviewed infants later diagnosed with Asperger's syndrome and saw a connection between early movement and AS. Children in the study showed delays or differences in crawling, walking, sitting, and the ability to right themselves. Some of the children used their right leg first when crawling and their left leg first when walking. Some babies seemed stuck in position when lying on their sides instead of moving their bodies to roll over. All of the babies observed did not sit independently by 6 months, and one child did not use his arms to protect himself from falling when learning to walk.

If your child has gross and fine motor skills deficits, occupational and physical therapies help by developing a variety of exercises pinpointed to your child's weaknesses. For fine motor skills, an occupational therapist may …

- Work on hand-eye coordination by playing catch or kicking balls.
- Use dancing or swimming to help build strength and arm and leg coordination.
- Use playground equipment in a supervised and supported environment.

Another reason for difficulty with sports is hypotonia, a generalized muscle weakness that affects posture, movement, strength, and coordination. If your child has signs of hypotonia, a physical therapist can develop exercises that you and your child can do on a daily basis to strengthen muscles and improve coordination.

Sensory Sensitivities

Bruce looked so handsome as he walked out the door on picture day. His mom had bought a special outfit—black jeans, a white dress shirt, and a tie. It was so different than his usual attire. Every day Bruce wore a T-shirt, nylon basketball shorts, short white socks, and sneakers. Most mornings it took about 10 minutes to get the socks on right, so that he couldn't feel any of the seams. His T-shirts didn't have tags, and when he got a new one his mom had to wash it at least 10 times to make it soft enough to be comfortable.

But all of Bruce's classmates were getting dressed up for picture day, and he wanted to as well. School had barely been in session for an hour when the teacher called and asked his mom to bring Bruce's "normal" clothes. Bruce had taken off his shirt because he couldn't stand the starchy, stiff collar. He was jumpy and irritable because he said his pants were itchy, and he was walking around barefoot because the new shoes were uncomfortable.

> **The Doctor's Take** If your child has sensory sensitivities, avoid strong-smelling laundry soaps and fabric softeners. The smell in his clothes could cause irritation all day and can disrupt sleep if it is on his sheets and pillows.

Sensory sensitivities are common in children with AS. Besides the feel of clothing, other hypersensitivities include:

- Sensitive to textures; may not like sticky substances or being touched, especially when unexpected

- Only eats certain foods; gags on some foods; may vomit easily; often "picky" eaters

- Dislikes loud noises; may cover ears or cry; may say loud noises hurt; easily distracted by noises

- Smells odors others may not; avoids places with strong smells

- Often bothered by bright lights or certain colors

If your child is hypersensitive, chances are the sensitivity won't go away. Aspies can't adjust to tactile discomforts in the same way others can. For example, another child in Bruce's class may have found the stiff collar to be uncomfortable, but after he got involved in an activity, he forgot about the collar bothering him. Bruce, on the other hand, would not be able to concentrate on anything until the offending touch was removed. Your child may be hypersensitive to things you don't even think about, such as the air from a fan or the buzzing of fluorescent lights.

Sensitivities can also be calming, for example, a child may rock back and forth or finger a piece of clothing. This movement or touch helps him relax and calm down in times of stress. Observe your child to find out what sensory stimuli is upsetting and which help your child calm down. Use relaxing stimuli, such as soft music or massage, to help manage stressful situations.

The Link Between Sensory Issues and Anxiety

MISC.

A study completed by Miriam Liss and others in 2005 showed that sensory sensitivities are linked to increased anxiety, including social anxiety disorder. This could be because of the need to avoid harm—for example, a sensitivity to touch can lead an Aspie to avoid close contact with others.

Although parents may initially fight a child's sensitivities, insisting he wear "appropriate" clothing or eat what is on his plate at dinner, this rarely works. The following are some tips for parents on dealing with such sensitivities:

- Accept sensitivities to clothing. Take your child to the store and let him pick out the clothing that is comfortable, as long as they are appropriate to the circumstances and season. He may prefer certain fabrics or items without tags. Bringing him along helps you find clothes he feels comfortable wearing.

- Experiment with a variety of foods with different colors and textures and allow him to try different foods. For example, a child may not like the texture of apples but may eat applesauce.

- Give your child something with a pleasant smell, such as a lavender sachet that he can hold close to his nose when he is around strong odors.

- Have earplugs on hand when going to events that may be noisy.

Occupational therapists help children with AS deal with hypersensitivities as well as reinforce motor skill development. Talk to your doctor or pediatrician about having your child assessed for hypersensitivities and ask for referrals to therapists who can work with your child.

Essential Takeaways

- Early detection and intervention increases your child's ability to learn appropriate behaviors and social skills.

- Children with AS may want to make friends but lack the social skills to know how to make friends.

- Rigid, literal thinking is one of the main signs of AS.

- Although no developmental delays in speech occur, children with AS have some language development concerns, such as not using inflection or sounding like a robot.

- Deficiencies in motor skills in infants and babies may help in early detection of AS.

chapter 3

Asperger's Syndrome in Girls

Why girls are diagnosed with AS less often than boys

How symptoms of AS manifest in girls

Special considerations of AS during puberty

Tips for parents on relationships and dating

Girls can and do have Asperger's syndrome (AS). Much like ADHD, which was considered a male disorder for many years, the medical community saw AS as a boy's condition. Today it is estimated that only one tenth to one quarter of those diagnosed with AS are girls. Experts believe girls with AS frequently fall under the radar, never receiving a diagnosis or getting the appropriate attention.

Obstacles to Diagnosis

Girls are known for being able to express emotions and are less likely to act out or be disruptive when frustrated or overwhelmed. Girls are usually quieter and more passive than boys at the same age. Parents and medical professionals often see girls as simply shy, overlooking possible symptoms of AS. Those who act out or act aggressively may be diagnosed sooner because these types of behaviors garner more attention from parents and teachers. Experts believe this is because these types of behaviors are more unusual in girls.

As you may have guessed, much of the criteria for diagnosing AS are based on how it manifests in boys. Doctors are not always familiar with how symptoms differ in girls. Special interests, for example, are often different. Boys with AS are frequently interested in topics involving science or transportation, such as weather or trains. Girls' special interests typically involve more mainstream topics like animals or classic literature. These interests do not draw as much attention because so many little girls love dogs, horses, or other animals. But these interests are much more intense or narrowly focused and often follow a girl into her teen years, long past when other girls have moved on to make-up and boys.

Moreover, symptoms usually appear milder in girls. Parents are sometimes more hesitant to bring daughters in for an evaluation, and doctors may believe the little girl will "grow out of it" as she matures. The degree of motor impairment in girls is usually less severe than in boys. Generally girls have a broader range of interests, and girls with AS seem to have a stronger desire to make emotional connections with other children and adults. According to Tony Attwood, author of *The Complete Guide to Asperger's Syndrome,* girls are more motivated to learn and are quicker to understand key concepts as compared to boys.

Research on Gender Differences in AS

MISC.

Two unpublished reports were presented at the 2006 International Meeting for Autism. One study completed at South Carolina and Duke Universities showed boys were more inattentive and more easily distracted than girls. The other study, completed at the University of Connecticut, observed girls with AS as toddlers and found they used pointing and pretend play more often than boys. They also followed an adult's gaze more often.

Fortunately, acceptance that girls can and do have Asperger's syndrome is growing. Women who have grown up without a diagnosis and now can put a label on their differences are speaking out. Books such as *Pretending to Be Normal* by Liane Holliday Willey and *Finding a Different Kind of Normal: Misadventures with Asperger Syndrome* by Jeannette Purkis tell the stories of these women. Clinical data, reported by doctors treating young girls, is reaching the medical community at large and the public.

Research, although slow, is beginning to include girls in studies about AS. As doctors and specialists understand more about how AS looks in girls, we will be better able to identify and treat girls at a younger age.

The Feminine Side of AS

In the following list of behaviors, you will see a number of similarities with how symptoms appear in boys. These symptoms are usually more subtle and harder for you as parents to notice. Many parents, however, indicate they knew something was "different" from the time the girls were babies or toddlers. Some have searched for answers for years, only to be told a daughter had obsessive compulsive disorder (OCD), anxiety, or was just shy. Parents accept the quirky behavior as "just part of their daughter's personality" because they have grown accustomed to their child's needs and communication style. As more and more is learned, it is now clear that distinct differences exist in how AS shows up in girls versus boys.

Young girls with AS lack reciprocity in play. Girls may appear as controlling, insisting on playing in a certain way, and ignoring requests to change the rules of a game. They may play with dolls by having them "act out" scenes from television shows, movies, or books. Any deviation from the script they create causes distress. They have a hard time including other girls in play because they may want to change the outcome or make up new scenarios and not play with such rigid structure.

Organization replaces pretend play. Aspies may arrange dolls in alphabetical order or by the color of their hair. They may organize accessories and categorize dolls and other toys. For them, this is play, and they find it relaxing and enjoyable. Aspies' playmates find this type of play boring and unimaginative and eventually might stop playing together.

Girls often become people pleasers. Many Aspies like order and structure and shy away from conflict. Girls with AS often go out of their way to keep their lives peaceful, acting in ways that minimize disruption to their routines.

Girls often use intelligence to hide social deficiencies. Girls mirror the mannerisms and actions of other girls, put a permanent smile on their faces, and try to look like they fit in, even though they are totally confused about what is going on in social situations. Aspies "study" other girls to mimic mannerisms, behaviors, and dress codes in order to adapt their styles to those around them.

Differences in Assessment of Girls

One of the criticisms of the current diagnostic criteria for AS is that it centers on behaviors commonly seen in boys. It does not take girls' behavior into account and doesn't give any guidelines or references to how these same symptoms manifest in girls. In the *Handbook of Behavioral and Emotional Problems* (Koenig and Tsatsanis, 2005), the authors offer suggestions on assessing girls for possible AS:

> The Doctor's Take
>
> Girls with AS, especially in the teen years, can develop an anxiety disorder or depression that makes diagnosis even more difficult.

- Referrals for services and treatments should be given even if the child comes close to meeting criteria for AS. This is because the original criteria were based on how AS shows up in boys, and girls may have milder symptoms.

- Medical providers should understand that signs of AS in girls may develop over time, specifically when girls enter adolescence.

- Communication skills and behaviors should not be compared to boys with AS but should be compared to communication and behaviors of other girls at that age.

- The assessment should take into account typical gender differences in socialization, communication, and behavior and societal or cultural expectations.

- Medical providers should consider that girls frequently do not exhibit the same level of repetitive behaviors and restricted interests that boys with AS do.

- The evaluation should take into account that girls with AS do not normally exhibit the same level of disruptive behaviors as boys with AS.

In addition, girls who are high-functioning are often able to answer questions about social situations because they have spent time observing and studying behaviors in people around them. They may take more time to process the question and form their answers. The answer, as well as the amount of time to answer, should be considered during the evaluation. The extra time needed to respond shows that although girls with AS may have a surface-level understanding of social situations and social norms, these Aspies do not have the in-depth understanding needed to quickly respond to questions. Direct observation of them in social situations with peers is the best way for a professional to assess these issues, but unfortunately this is not always possible.

The Adolescent Aspie

Boys have more problems socially in the younger years, but girls struggle more socially when they reach adolescence and the teen years. When a girl is young, she sometimes has a single friend or a small group of friends who nurture or mother her, helping her through social situations, comforting her when upset. But when she reaches adolescence, social situations become much harder to navigate.

Adapting to Changes During Puberty

Puberty is a hard time for all girls, but it is much more difficult for girls with AS. Your child probably resists change of any kind, and the changes occurring during puberty are no exception. The beginning of menstruation, changes in the shape of her body, and new types of social interactions are all scary. She is frightened, confused, and frustrated because no matter how much she fights it, changes in her body continue to happen.

For you as parents, talking about topics such as body changes, relationships, and sex is difficult, but your daughter isn't going to know what is going on unless you explain it. You will need to teach about the nuances of love, dating, relationships, and sexuality and what constitutes appropriate and inappropriate behavior—both your daughter's behavior and her potential partner's behavior. You may feel your daughter is too young for this information, but by the time she reaches puberty, you should have already laid the foundation. Now your conversations should build on her understanding of more mature relationships. One myth about children with autism and AS is that they don't have any interest or emotional capacity for love relationships, but this is not true. It is better to feel uncomfortable now than to leave your daughter unprepared later.

> **Aspie Advice**
>
> Relationship circles are a good way to explain different relationships. Begin by creating a small circle and continue drawing larger circles around the first one. The innermost circle represents your family. In the outer circles, list relatives, acquaintances, friends, best friends, opposite-sex friends, boyfriends. In each circle write the types of behaviors and conversation topics that are appropriate for that group. Include appropriate greetings, such as a hug or a handshake, and what topics should not be discussed.

As your daughter's body changes, it is a good time to talk about how she needs to respond to those changes. Nutrition and exercise become more important. Showering and hygiene are often a problem for girls with AS. She might not like to get wet and doesn't understand the need for daily showers. Due to sensory sensitivities, she may find it uncomfortable to wear a bra, use deodorant, or use different soaps and lotions. You may need to find unscented and hypoallergenic body products. You may find beginning with a sports bra helps introduce your daughter to the constricting feeling of bras. It's best to start this process early to allow your daughter extra time to adjust.

You also need to prepare your daughter for getting her period. Although this may be uncomfortable, you should practice what your daughter should do, including how to attach a pad to her panties and how often pads should be changed. Many books are available on this topic. If your daughter is a reader, she might prefer to read them alone first. You can follow up the books by having a discussion on what changes your daughter can expect to happen over the next few years. If your daughter doesn't like to read, choose a quiet time to go through a book together. Although these changes are scary for your daughter, preparing her for what is going to happen helps.

Unfortunately, not much information is available about how hormonal changes affect AS symptoms. Keeping a calendar throughout the month to track how she feels during the entire cycle helps her know what to expect, both physically and emotionally. When does she start to feel PMS? How long does her period last? What other symptoms is she having? How does her mood change? The more you and your daughter know about the entire cycle, the more you can create routines and manage stress.

Navigating the Teen Years

The teen years open up a whole new set of difficulties for girls with AS. Your daughter may have been able to keep up socially with younger girls, where social interactions revolved more around activities than around conversation. In the teen years all of this changes, and your daughter could have a hard time keeping up with the nuances of how teen girls talk and bond with each other. At this age girls are expected to share thoughts, ideas, and feelings and to listen as their friends share theirs.

Changing Friendships

MISC.

Mary and Cindy were best friends. They were together in school, the Girl Scouts, and soccer teams. Their friendship began to change when Cindy started talking about "girl" things such as boys, the future, and relationships. When Cindy talked about her hopes and fears, Mary looked at her blankly, listened for a few minutes, and then went back to familiar topics. Mary felt hurt when Cindy told her that she had a new best friend. Mary's parents were concerned she was showing signs of depression and took her for an evaluation. She was diagnosed with both depression and AS.

Aspies are sometimes more sensitive to criticism than other young people. Wanting to please others, they see this criticism as something they did "wrong" and try to find ways to correct the behavior. Your daughter may mimic others by adopting their mannerisms, how they speak, and their facial expressions. She may take on different identities in an effort to be socially accepted. Or your daughter may instead become more withdrawn and anxious, avoiding social situations and spending all her time alone.

Girls with AS frequently wear clothes that are loose fitting and do not match what the other girls their age are wearing. Those with sensory sensitivities wear clothes that offer comfort. Your daughter might not see the purpose of fashionable clothes, instead opting for practical clothes. Some parents find it helpful to talk with other parents, window-shop at the mall, and browse on the internet to find out what types of clothes other teens are wearing. Usually there is enough variety to find clothes that meet your daughter's needs but won't make her stand out. It may be helpful to take your daughter shopping or to bring home a number of different outfits to let her try on in private. After you have an idea of what your daughter likes, you can purchase stylish clothes that allow her to feel comfortable.

When they are young, girls with AS can have imaginary friends, and this can continue into the teen years. These imaginary friends help your daughter create a world where she is accepted exactly as she is. This feeling of acceptance as well as creating a world where she feels secure and safe is often misunderstood. Medical professionals may see this type of behavior as hallucinations or delusions and misdiagnose a teen girl with AS as having schizophrenia or another type of mental illness.

Parents play an important role in helping their Aspies navigate all the changes in a teen's social life. Following are some tips to help:

- Be specific when giving instructions and be prepared to state instructions several times.

- Understand that being able to repeat instructions does not necessarily mean that your daughter understood what the instructions mean.

- As you give your daughter more responsibility and chores around the house, break down chores into small tasks.

- Use *multisensory* approaches to teaching different skills and for creating schedules.

- Role-play different social scenarios; take turns with you modeling appropriate behaviors and then allowing your daughter to play-act.

- Write social scripts for things like talking on the phone, meeting someone, asking for help, or inviting someone to your house.

- Look for social groups that revolve around your daughter's interests or groups of other teens with AS where she will feel comfortable and can practice social skills. Look for online groups of girls with AS if none are in your area.

- Teach relaxation strategies such as deep breathing, keeping a diary, self-talk, yoga, and daily exercise.

> **Definition**
>
> **Multisensory** approaches incorporate two or more of the senses during the learning process. For example, when giving instructions, say them out loud, act out a portion of the instruction, write them down, and include pictures. By using several different senses, you increase your daughter's ability to comprehend and remember the instructions.

Another idea to help your daughter be more aware of nonverbal language in others is to watch movies together, turning off the sound and discussing what the characters may be feeling based on body language alone and making predictions on what the characters will do next. Then turn the sound back on and listen to tone of voice. You can also videotape your daughter in various social situations. Play back the video, discussing what she did right and what she could do differently.

Girls with AS usually have a higher interest in social connections and relationships than boys with AS, even though they may not possess the social skills to form and participate in the complex relationships of the teen years. Some prefer not to worry about friends, finding social interaction too difficult and exhausting. Some are happy with just one friend. Make sure you are respecting your daughter's wants. As parents we have different ideas of friendship and push those ideas on our child. Provide opportunities for social interaction but don't pressure your daughter to create friendships if she is not ready.

Your daughter might prefer to spend time with boys rather than girls. Some experts talk about AS as being "Hyper-Maleness." Core aspects of AS are lower social awareness, lack of intuition on emotional issues, heightened analytical skills or focus, facts being more important than feelings, and an overemphasis on being "right," all traits attributed more to males than females. Girls who demonstrate these skills are viewed as more aggressive, more "businesslike," or other less flattering things. Because generally less demand exists for the more advanced social skills in boys' relationships, your daughter might find it easier to be around boys.

Focus on Relationships

One of the most stressful times in a parent's life is when her daughter is ready to start dating, even more so if your daughter has AS. Your daughter may be socially awkward, or she may be socially unaware. Unfortunately, this can leave her open to being used by boys and even abused by sexual predators. She may misinterpret social signals, assuming someone is interested in her when he is not. She may want a physical and emotional connection and be desperate to have a boyfriend, willing to do whatever the boy wants. This is more difficult for parents to practice because opportunities involve actual social situations.

> **The Doctor's Take**
>
> Parents should be aware of the warning signs of abuse. Pay attention to unexplained bruises, torn or missing clothes, avoidance of certain people or places, withdrawal, depression, self-mutilation, or changes in sleeping patterns. If you suspect a date or someone else is abusing your daughter, ask questions and, if needed, contact the police department to file a report.

As with friendships, some girls may not be interested in romantic relationships. As a parent, you should respect your daughter's choice but be ready if she reaches a point when she changes her mind. If your daughter is interested in dating, she may need extra help in understanding how romantic relationships work—for example, you might explain how friendships and romantic relationships are different. Her first experience with flirting might be confusing for her, and you can help by talking about what it feels like to be attracted to someone and what the signs are that someone is interested in her and how teenagers commonly show these feelings. You will also need to teach specific dating skills, such as:

- What should happen on a first date, second date, and so on

- The right to say "no" if she does not want to go on a date with someone and the right to go out on one date and not want to go on a second

- What constitutes appropriate behavior on a date (both her behavior and her date's behavior) and what to do if her date acts inappropriately, such as yelling "no," saying "no" loudly, and using specific body language to show she is uncomfortable

- How to set boundaries, privacy rules, and the difference between questions and demands

- How to end the date, both when it has gone well and when it has not gone well

As your daughter starts dating, you need to help with everything from getting ready for the date to what to do when the date is over. In the beginning you may feel more comfortable with dates that consist of a few teens going out together or having you or another responsible adult chaperone. Although many teens object to their parents coming on a date, you can get around this by inviting the date to your house for dinner or having an older cousin or neighbor join your daughter on her date.

Having one or two dates is different than being in a relationship, and your daughter will continue to need your help understanding the dynamics and different stages of a relationship. Discuss what normally happens as a relationship progresses. Let your daughter know you are available to answer all her questions, but accept that she may feel uncomfortable talking about sexual matters with you. If this happens, have a list of several trusted adults she can talk to, especially if there are warning signs of an unhealthy relationship. Every teen experiences rejection at some time, and your daughter is probably not going to be an exception. When talking about dating, discuss what traits and characteristics your daughter finds important in a boyfriend. Help her to understand that everyone looks for something different, and she might be attracted to someone who is not attracted to her. Help her develop coping strategies for dealing with rejection.

Developing Independence

During the teen years, your daughter's classmates will be gaining more and more independence from their parents, taking steps toward their future, and talking about college, careers, and marriage. You might be wondering whether your daughter will ever be able to make it on her own or if she will always need assistance. Many adult Aspies do live independent lives, and the skills you teach your daughter throughout her life will help prepare her. But executive function deficits cause problems with future planning.

> **Aspie Advice**
>
> Independent skills include understanding what behaviors are considered appropriate while alone but not accepted in public. For example, your daughter might not realize that using certain hygiene products, burping, and scratching in private areas requires privacy.

Help your daughter to gain self-awareness. This means helping her to realize what her strengths are, what she does well, and what type of person she is. You can create lists of words describing what you see as your daughter's strengths and abilities and ask her to choose the ones she would use. Other parents create a poster board with a picture and let their daughter write words around the picture. Include pictures of activities your daughter enjoys and what she thinks she would like to do as she gets older.

Make a list of skills your daughter can currently do without assistance, such as dressing, showering, and completing homework. Create a second list of independent skills your daughter has not yet mastered. Choose one item on the list at a time and work together to conquer that skill. Create opportunities for your daughter to succeed and make sure to give her feedback. Your comments need to be honest and encouraging but not critical.

Essential Takeaways

- Because girls are usually better at expressing emotions and less likely to act disruptive, symptoms of AS can be overlooked.
- The current diagnostic criteria are based on how symptoms manifest in boys. The medical community is still learning how symptoms manifest in girls.
- Although boys have more difficulty with social skills when young, girls experience more problems in social skills in preteen and teen years.
- Girls with AS are at risk for being used in relationships because they can misinterpret social signals.

chapter 4

Related Conditions

Helping AS children deal with anxiety

Comparing AS and obsessive compulsive disorder

How depression shows up in children with AS

Problems associated with sensory sensitivities

A number of medical conditions are common in individuals with Asperger's syndrome (AS). Some of these share similar symptoms and make the diagnostic process confusing. Others are seen with a higher frequency in Aspies than in the general public. In this chapter, we look at some of the most common co-existing, or comorbid, conditions with AS.

Anxiety Disorders

Children with AS can excessively worry about social performance. Their confusion about the world around them, their desire to fit in, and consistent worry about making a mistake in public can, and often does, develop into an anxiety disorder. Because Aspies need structure and routine to feel secure, changes—especially those that are unexpected—can cause anxiety.

Anxiety disorders are characterized by consistent worry that is disproportionate to the situation. For example, most children are nervous about an upcoming test at school but if your child has anxiety, he may worry for days or weeks prior to the test. He might lose sleep, feel physically sick, and even find reasons to not go to school on the day of the test. This heightened sense of dread and worry could signal an anxiety disorder.

> **The Doctor's Take**
>
> Differences exist between stress and anxiety as well as differences between worry and an anxiety disorder. Events, both good and bad, can cause stress. The same event can result in completely different reactions for each person. For example, at a wedding, the stress level for the mother of the bride and the best man is different. How we adapt to stress is a part of the learning process, but when we do not adapt well to our stress, we may be talking about an anxiety disorder.

All children with anxiety can appear agitated, irritable, and tense and may avoid activities that bring on these feelings. The following are additional ways a child with AS may show signs of anxiety:

- Restlessness; unable to relax or calm down

- Tendency to *ruminate*

- Requesting that you confirm the same information over and over

- An increase in routines and rituals as a way to bring order into their lives

- Becoming more rigid in thinking

- Spending more time with a special interest and using it as a way to escape situations that invoke anxiety

- Regressing to earlier behaviors that you thought they had outgrown

> **Definition**
>
> To **ruminate** is to think deeply about a subject, to turn it over and over in the mind beyond that which is typical under similar circumstances.

You can help your child develop stress management and coping techniques to help reduce anxiety. Some common ways of decreasing nervousness are:

Relaxation strategies. Create a quiet place in your home and ask teachers to have an area of the classroom where your child can escape to when feeling anxious. This area should be free of social and conversational requirements and be visually calming. You can also teach your child deep-breathing techniques, meditation, and guided imagery as ways to help calm their thoughts.

Divert attention. Help your child find an activity that is not frustrating or is easily completed but is one that he enjoys. This can be related to your child's special interest or could be another activity he enjoys, such as watching a video or spending time on the computer.

Exercise. Physical exercise tends to reduce anxiety immediately, and daily exercise programs reduce anxiety throughout the day. Teach your child to take a walk (with your permission) or have a set exercise routine for your child to use either every day or when he is feeling overwhelmed.

Sleep. Help your child get the right amount and type of sleep he needs. Research indicates significant decreases occur in the level of anxiety a person experiences with positive changes in sleep patterns. Sleep is a natural restorative and can significantly aid in reducing stress. The amount of sleep required changes as we age, and people mistakenly believe that it consistently gets less as we grow older. In fact, teenagers often require more sleep than tweens do, with the need going back up to 9 to 10 hours per night on average during those stressful teen years.

In school, request not only a special area in the classroom but also times throughout the day your child can go to the library or have set times of the day to leave the classroom. Your child and teacher can have a secret signal for times when anxious feelings are heightened. The teacher can take steps to help relieve stress, maybe by giving the child a note to bring to the office.

For many children, these stress-management techniques will help reduce anxiety symptoms. However, if despite your efforts, anxiety levels are still high and interfering with your child's ability to function in everyday activities, he may need additional help and treatment. This can include therapy and medication.

Aspie Advice
Help prepare your child for situations and events that are stressful. Discuss settings, triggers, and what actions he can take. Role-play scenarios and plan out social scripts to help reduce anxiety in new situations.

Cognitive behavioral therapy (CBT) has been found to be effective in treating anxiety. This type of treatment changes the way a person thinks and reacts to stimuli. It can include exposure or desensitization exercises. One example is a child who is afraid of dogs. A therapist starts by guiding a child to think about a dog, while relaxed. After he has mastered thinking about the dog without anxiety, the therapist has him look at pictures of dogs or brings a dog into the office, but the dog stays on the other side of the room. The therapist slowly bridges the distance between the child and the dog. Each step can take several weeks, but eventually it reduces or eliminates the child's fear of dogs. Some Aspies have a hard time relating an experience to different locations, so the therapist may need to introduce dogs in a variety of locations, such as in the office, outside at the park, and at home.

Obsessive Compulsive Disorder

Obsessive compulsive disorder (OCD) is a type of anxiety disorder characterized by obsessive, intrusive thoughts and compulsions, tasks, or rituals, which are done over and over in an effort to reduce or stop the obsessions. Because Aspies often complete certain rituals, such as lining up toys in a certain way, and are obsessed with a special interest, it is sometimes confusing when determining whether a child has OCD or AS, but there are specific differences. A certain level of obsessive and compulsive behaviors is seen as typical in people with AS and does not necessarily indicate the need for another diagnosis.

Obsessions are recurrent and persistent thoughts, impulses, or images that are intrusive and are accompanied with stress or anxiety. Compulsions, strong impulses to perform an act, are used to neutralize the obsessions. An example of OCD obsessions and compulsions is the fear of germs. A person continually washes her hands in an effort to reduce the fear of germs, sometimes to the point of having red, dry, chapped hands. Someone with OCD often realizes her obsessions are "in the mind" but feels helpless to end them and helpless to stop the behavior.

Aspies are sometimes diagnosed with OCD, but their obsessions and compulsions must not be caused by their rigid thinking and must be different from prior behaviors. For example, your child might previously have needed to spend time interacting with his passion, but you recently have noticed this need become much more urgent, to the point where he becomes angry or agitated when told it is time to stop and come to the dinner table. OCD behaviors also must interfere with daily functioning, such as not getting homework done because he must check his bedroom over and over to ensure toys are still lined up correctly or needs to repeatedly wash his hands. If you begin to notice these types of behaviors, you may want to talk to your doctor. Other behaviors to watch for include:

- Physical actions that seem out of your child's control, or he tells you, "I can't help it, I have to do this"

- Loses sleep because activities continue to "require" more and more time, refuses to participate in other activities, or ignores responsibilities in order to perform actions or rituals

- Doesn't want to do anything else because rituals and actions have become all-consuming

The Doctor's Take

When talking to your doctor about OCD, it is important to explain how behaviors have changed. List examples of previous behaviors and current behaviors. Because some traits of Asperger's syndrome can be similar to OCD, it is important to notice the changes in behaviors.

OCD can be treated with medications and/or therapy. If you believe your child is showing signs of OCD, take the time to document behaviors, including when and how often your child completes actions and rituals, and discuss with his doctor. Remember, if your child does have OCD, the behaviors are a result of a medical condition and are not done to annoy you.

Attention Deficit Hyperactivity Disorder

Attention Deficit Hyperactivity Disorder (ADHD) and Asperger's syndrome are two separate and distinct conditions. Like OCD, some similar or shared symptoms can be identified, but so can differences. Some medical professionals believe that children should be screened for both conditions so treatment plans can target problem behaviors more effectively. ADHD is treated in the United States primarily with medication, but the National Institute of Mental Health consensus reports indicate that medication plus behavior therapy strategies are more effective. However, research by Luke Tsai, MD, indicates that those with AS do not typically respond to medications routinely found effective for ADHD in the same way that those with ADHD respond to those same medications.

The Doctor's Take

The DSM strongly discourages diagnosing ADHD in children with AS. Some doctors see ADHD everywhere and diagnose the two together, but often the "symptoms" of ADHD are part of the AS. In some cases both are present independently of each other, but this is considered rare by those not selling a medication or pushing a "cure" for one or both.

Both children with ADHD and with AS can hyperfocus when involved in an activity they are highly interested in but are inattentive when working on an activity that does not hold much interest. Both have a hard time shifting attention to a new activity, although children with AS do this because of a need to complete one activity before starting another. Both have poor social skills, although for different reasons. Children with ADHD do not always play well with other children, but this is typically because of impulsivity. They want social interaction and know how to play, but symptoms of ADHD interfere with how well they play. Children with ADHD also have a wide range of interests and do not typically have problems with communication.

Despite the differences, some behavioral strategies work well for both children with ADHD and children with Asperger's:

- Minimizing distractions and offering a quiet place to play or study

- Breaking assignments or chores into small tasks

- Highlighting relevant information

- Providing consistency through structure and routine

Both children with ADHD and with AS can have sensory sensitivities and problems with motor skills, although neither of these aspects are used to diagnose ADHD.

Depression

The causes of depression, especially in Aspies, are not clear. While depression is thought to be, at least in part, hereditary, it can also occur because of environmental factors. Some studies, including one by Kim Tatum, show that anywhere from 15 percent to 33 percent of individuals with AS also have symptoms of depression. Although most believe the hallmark symptom of depression is sadness, in children and adolescents the predominant emotion also can be irritability.

Aspies often want and crave emotional connections and friends; they want to be liked and accepted; and they want to be like their peers. The effort to fit in is exhausting and emotionally draining. As your child continues to try and fail, he begins to believe he is socially defective. Because the very nature of depression includes believing that the worst possible outcome is unavoidable, children may believe that things will never get better, that they will always be unhappy social outcasts.

Symptoms of depression may appear as the following:

- Sadness or irritability lasting more than two weeks and not attributed to a specific event, such as the death of a family member where sadness is expected

- Whining; moaning; clingy behavior; needing constant reassurance

- Decreased interest in special interests; may pass up opportunities to participate in favorite activities

- Fascination with morbid thoughts, stating "No one loves me" or "No one wants me"

- Increased agitation or irritability

- Excessively tired; acts like it is a great effort to move

- Changes in eating habits—could be a loss of appetite or eating too much

- Changes in sleep pattern, either increases or decreases

The Cycle of Depression

MISC.

Depression can lead to a vicious cycle. Because of the depression, your child withdraws socially. Because of the social withdrawal, fewer opportunities are available to practice social skills, which results in an even deeper social withdrawal. If you see signs of depression, seek help and look for safe, secure places for your child to practice social skills, such as AS support groups.

You may not readily notice depression because a child with AS has a difficult time expressing emotion. He may not be able to tell you he feels sad or even understand what is going on, becoming withdrawn instead. If you notice your child's special interests taking on a morbid tone, such as a preoccupation with death, he may be trying to communicate how he is feeling.

Depression is usually treated with therapy and medication, but it is important to find someone who is knowledgeable about AS as well as depression. The two best researched therapy treatments for depression are interpersonal therapy and CBT. CBT focuses on altering dysfunctional thought patterns in order to improve emotion and increase more functional behaviors. This approach seems incredibly well suited to the interpersonal and learning style of Aspies.

Learning Disabilities

Learning disabilities are separate and distinct disorders from AS, even though the two share characteristics. Finding a specialist who understands the differences is important so you have an accurate diagnosis and can, together with teachers and medical professionals, select the strategies that will best help your child succeed. The following sections explain a few of the learning disabilities that share symptoms with AS.

Disorder of Written Expression

Aspies frequently have problems with written expression, also known as dysgraphia. This condition is characterized by poor writing skills caused by weaknesses in fine motor control, conceptualizing, and preorganizing material. Although common in children with dyslexia, this disorder is a writing disorder and occurs regardless of reading ability.

If your child has dysgraphia, she may lack basic spelling skills, have difficulty with letter reversals (p and q, b and d), or write the wrong word
when putting her thoughts on paper. Her writing may be crammed
together, without spaces between words and sentences. She may also make
frequent errors in spelling, punctuation, and grammar. With many Aspies,
handwriting is sloppy and sometimes illegible. Using a keyboard or text-
to-speech software is helpful and sometimes necessary.

Nonverbal Learning Disorder

Nonverbal learning disorder (NVLD) is characterized by early language
acquisition and speech development. Children with NVLD often have a
large vocabulary and are considered "auditory learners." They typically
have difficulty with nonverbal memory, executive functions, mathematical
reasoning, reading comprehension, and handwriting. Those with NVLD
are usually less active and don't physically explore their environment.
They have problems with tasks requiring nonverbal memory skills and
executive functioning.

> **Aspie Advice**
>
> Children with NVLD and/or AS benefit from clear, concise, step-by-step
> directions. When giving instructions, state your expectations first. Avoid
> jargon, double-meanings, and sarcasm.

Both children with AS and those with NVLD have problems with social
interactions because of their inability to read nonverbal social cues, such
as body language, facial expressions, and tone of voice. Both may have
problems forming close emotional relationships with others, although
this is sometimes missed in children with NVLD until late childhood or
adolescence. Other similarities between Asperger's syndrome and NVLD
include the following:

- Problems with motor skills, especially balance, coordination, and
  fine motor skills

- Resistance to change

- Sensory issues

- Difficulty processing tactile and visual-spatial information

There are also a number of differences between NVLD and AS:

Imaginative play. Children with AS do not normally engage in imaginative play but children with NVLD do not lack imaginative play.

Uses toys for intended purposes. Children with NVLD typically use toys for the purpose they were made for; children with AS frequently use toys for different purposes.

Language. While children with AS have difficulty sharing ideas and thoughts, children with NVLD will use language skills to share ideas with others.

Sensory Integration Disorder

Sensory integration disorder (SID), also known as sensory processing disorder, is when a person has difficulty processing sensory information and appropriately responding to it. Aspies often find sensory problems more difficult to manage than social deficiencies. Hyposensitivity refers to showing little or no reaction to stimulus, such as not feeling hot or cold. In hypersensitivity, stimulus, even a light touch or a bright light, can be any-where from bothersome to painful. Aspies frequently show signs of being hypo- and hypersensitive, sometimes changing from one to the other within minutes. Hypersensitivity, however, tends to be more prevalent and presents more difficulties.

All senses—auditory, smell, taste, visual, and touch—can cause problems, but your child may be more sensitive in one area than in another.

MISC.

Sensory Distractions

Billy was identified with AS in elementary school, had various supports through elementary school, and was now mainstreamed. In middle school, he became irritable and distracted. ADHD was suggested; Billy was pre-scribed a stimulant, but he became hostile and belligerent. His parents stopped the stimulant, and his behaviors subsided, but the original symp-toms remained. Upon further investigation it was discovered that Billy was sitting next to a laser printer in both his classrooms. These machines emit-ted a hum. When the machines were removed, Billy's distractibility and irritability decreased.

Auditory

According to one study completed by Steven M. Bromley, MD, anywhere from 70 percent to 85 percent of Aspies have auditory sensitivities. Several different types of sounds are disturbing to people with auditory sensitivities:

- Loud, unexpected, or unpredictable sounds cause the most problems—dogs barking, people yelling, telephones ringing, babies crying, and sirens

- High-pitched continuous sounds such as small electric motors in a blender or vacuum cleaner

- Complex sounds that are difficult to interpret such as being in a large, noisy crowd

To help your child, offer ear plugs and have him listen to music through headphones. It also helps to make others aware of the sensitivity to minimize sudden noises and reduce background sounds as much as possible.

Taste and Smell

Children with sensitivities to smell can frequently detect odors that other people cannot. Many find certain smells distasteful, especially strong foods, perfumes, or toiletries. Your child may run away or leave the room when confronted with certain smells, not able to explain why the smell bothers him. Both the texture and taste of food also trigger food sensitivities. Your child might have a restricted diet because of these sensitivities, eating only one or two foods and wanting the foods to be cooked in the same way each time. He may gag or vomit if tastes or textures are bothersome.

As a parent, you might worry whether your child is getting the proper nutrition if his taste and smell sensitivities have severely limited his diet. Most children grow out of this type of sensitivity by the time puberty is reached or in the teen years. But if it is a concern, talk with a dietician to help create a nutritious diet.

Visual

Many Aspies, although not all, are visual learners. Parents and teachers are encouraged to use visual cues to help reinforce different concepts or to help those children struggling with reading. You might consider pictures to be very effective tools to facilitate communication. However, for those with visual sensitivities, too much visual stimuli can cause *sensory overload,* overwhelming your child. Imagine going to the mall during the holiday season, with bright lights, decorations, and lots of people. Your child can quickly become overstimulated from all of the visual details.

Definition

Sensory overload is when one or more of the senses is strained and makes it difficult to focus on the task at hand. Sensory overload can often result in meltdowns or tantrums.

Bright lights, especially fluorescent lights that flicker, can be painful for those with visual sensitivities. Many times the flickering of these lights is not noticeable to others, but for those with sensitivities, bright lights are difficult to be around. Sun glare in the classroom or when driving in the car can be distracting or even painful. Offer your child sunglasses and ask the teacher to seat your child away from the window or to use blinds to reduce sun glare.

Touch

We normally think of being touched as a pleasant sensation, but for those with sensory sensitivities, touch can be unbearable. If your child is sensitive to touch, he may avoid being with other children because he is afraid of being accidently touched. The head, upper arms, and palms are normally most sensitive to touch, which causes many children to dislike having their hair washed or their hair cut. As with sound, unpredictable or sudden touch is more difficult. When a child is young, friends, relatives and even strangers often reach out to touch or hug a child. Your child may want no part of this, crying, biting, or even hitting when touched. As a parent, you can request relatives not hug your child, showing respect for his personal space.

Clothes are another problem for many. Tags need to be cut out of clothes, and socks need to be put on just right to feel comfortable inside shoes. Some have described the feeling of certain clothes as flesh being rubbed with sandpaper. Many parents find that cotton and all-natural clothing is best. Although children without AS, even when wearing uncomfortable clothes, will be able to ignore the sensation and complete activities, your child may not be able to do so. Uncomfortable clothing will prevent him from paying attention to anything else.

Children with AS do not always have an aversion to touch. Some like hugs, to be wrapped in a cozy blanket, or massaged. It is important for parents to respect their child's needs; touches should be on your child's terms. Ask before giving a hug and let your child know it is okay to not want to be touched sometimes.

Seizures

One in four children with an autism spectrum disorder develops seizures. This can start in early childhood, but sometimes seizures appear in adolescence.

Aspie Advice	Many seizures do not require medical attention. An obvious exception would be if your child is injured during a seizure. And if a seizure lasts more than five minutes or one seizure quickly follows another, call for medical help. Always follow the advice of your child's pediatric neurologist.

General seizures can include convulsions or staring spells and are classified based on how large they are and whether you can easily see muscle movement during the seizure. If your child has a partial seizure, he may be able to sense movement or other sensations but may not be able to respond. He may be confused or disoriented, fumble, wander, or repeat words and phrases.

During some seizures, your child can appear to be staring at you but totally ignoring everything you say. You might not be aware that he is having seizures unless you are looking directly at his face. For some children, seizures may occur for a period of time before you notice something is wrong. Some of the signs your child is having seizures include the following.

- Your child's behavior regresses
- No forward progress is made in school or cognitive abilities
- Aggression or emotional outbursts occur

If you begin to notice these types of behaviors and cannot attribute them to your child's AS, or if they are a definite change from previous behaviors, you can talk to his doctor about the possibility of seizures.

Seizures can also occur during transitions to and from sleep. If your child has been dry through the night and suddenly is wetting the bed and looking "out of it" in the morning, he may need to be seen by a pediatric neurologist. Your child may need an EEG to confirm or rule out whether seizures are occurring.

Treatment for seizures includes anti-seizure medication. Parents can help by monitoring sleep, as a lack of sleep can trigger seizures; also make sure your child stays away from caffeine and minimize stress. If your child is on stimulant medication, talk with his doctor about whether the medication should be discontinued, as these medications can exacerbate seizures.

Essential Takeaways

- Aspies have a high risk of developing mental illnesses such as anxiety, depression, obsessive compulsive disorder, or Attention Deficit Hyperactivity Disorder.
- ADHD and AS share some symptoms, but these are two distinct conditions.
- Sensory sensitivities often cause more problems than social problems in Aspies.
- One in four children with autism spectrum disorders will develop seizures.

chapter 5

Treatment

Finding the right doctors

Seeking physical therapy for coordination problems

Applying behavioral strategies

Considering alternative treatments

No single treatment exists for Asperger's syndrome (AS). No medication takes away symptoms and no cure will make your child "normal." But many different methods can help strengthen your child's weaknesses and help her live a happy and productive life. The best treatment for AS is a "package deal." Your child's treatment team works together choosing a combination of therapies specific to her needs. The package for one Aspie is not necessarily appropriate for another Aspie. Because each person's AS manifests in a unique way, the treatment plan should also be unique. Any good treatment plan includes secondary diagnoses, such as anxiety or seizures. In this chapter, we review some of the components of a comprehensive treatment plan for AS.

Choosing a Treatment Team

Because your child's treatment consists of several different types of therapy, you need to create and work with a treatment team. Some of the different specialists include family doctor or pediatrician, psychologist, developmental pediatrician, neurologist, behavior analyst, physical and occupational therapists, speech language pathologist, social worker, psychiatrist, and nutritionist. Each team member works closely with you and your child and must communicate with the other team members. Your family doctor or pediatrician often works as the coordinator of the team, bringing information from various sources to create a complete picture of your child's strengths and weaknesses.

Aspie Advice

Keep a notebook that provides a chronological record of your child's evaluations and treatments. At the beginning of any appointment, give the notebook to the treatment provider, letting her see what other team members have written, and ask her to supply a summary of the day's treatment and concerns or improvements noted during the session.

You obviously want the best possible treatment for your child, and that means finding the best possible medical professionals. During your first contact with a provider, he asks many questions and completes an assessment of your child's current development. But you also have the right to ask questions. It is important for both you and your child to feel comfortable with the different therapists and doctors. Some potential questions for you to ask include:

- What type and extent of experience does the person have working with Aspies? Where is the work done with Aspies? Mostly in schools, offices, or in the home?

- Can this professional provide references from other parents? Previous supervisors?

- Does this person have updated background clearances? Can this person show you child-abuse clearance and criminal record checks?

- How are therapy sessions structured? Does this provider have video recordings of therapy sessions you can view? Can you observe a therapy session with another child? Is this provider willing to work one-on-one with your child as a "sample session" while you observe?

- How does this person normally communicate with other team members?

The Doctor's Take

When talking with a medical professional, be sure to ask what education she has received specific to AS. Find out whether she routinely attends conferences and seminars to keep up with new information and research findings.

Medical professionals and therapists should never exclude you from treatment sessions. In the beginning there may be a few sessions alone to get to know your child, but after that, you should always have the opportunity of observing therapy sessions. Therapy sessions should not contradict your family values. Because AS is not caused by a lack of parent-child bonding, therapists should not focus on the parent-child relationship except during family counseling sessions. If a therapist believes that simply fixing or strengthening your bond with your child will help improve behavior, find a different therapist.

All therapists and treatment team members should set goals for your child's progress. These goals need to be specific and measurable. For example, "improve social skills" is not a goal. "Be able to look someone in the eye when conversing" is a goal. Without concrete goals, you have no way of measuring whether a specific course of treatment is working. Many are broken down into small steps, allowing you, your child, and the therapist to see progress along the way.

It's possible your insurance coverage or referrals from county agencies limit your choices regarding who will be working with your child. Even so, you still have the right to request a second opinion or ask for a referral to a different provider if you are concerned about the level of care your child is receiving. Talk with your insurance company or a supervisor in your county program if you are unhappy with your current treatments.

Different Types of Therapy

Many different types of therapies are useful in helping Aspies become independent and live fulfilling lives. Finding the right therapists for your child is similar to going to a buffet with your family. Each person has his or her own favorite foods, and each plate looks different because it is based on individual tastes. Building a team of therapists works on the same concept. You work with the therapists who can best fill the needs of your unique child.

Physical and Occupational Therapy

Aspies are sometimes described as clumsy and uncoordinated. Their muscle tone is not as well developed, and their movements seem choppy. Aspies may be unbalanced and have trouble running, jumping, and swinging on swings or on the monkey bars. Physical therapy is often used to address these problems.

> **The Doctor's Take**
>
> It is sometimes difficult for a child to qualify for physical therapy if she is not physically disabled but "merely" clumsy. In those instances, you may want to look into enrolling your child in community programs for gymnastics, swimming, or other whole-body activities to help improve muscle tone and coordination.

The physical therapist initially evaluates your child to determine current abilities and challenges. Based on this, she develops a plan to target specific areas and increase motor skills that includes exercises, assisted movement, and, if needed, orthopedic devices. Generally, physical therapy is provided for 30 minutes to 1 hour at a time, once a week, with parents assisting in daily exercises. Some children may require more intense therapy programs several times per week.

Occupational therapists work on skills needed to function "at work." For children, these skills include play, chores, self-care, schoolwork, and fine motor skills. To help improve functioning in these areas, occupational therapists develop exercises and programs to work on cognitive, physical, and motor skills. Like the physical therapist, during the initial visit, the occupational therapist completes an assessment, but instead of focusing on just physical development, the occupational therapist looks at psychological, social, and environmental factors that are affecting your child's functioning.

Goals are developed based on your child's unique needs. Some examples include:

- Independent dressing and self-care, such as grooming and eating
- Increasing fine motor skills, such as holding a pencil correctly
- Learning to transition from one activity to another

- Developing play skills to help develop complex social skills

- Breaking large tasks into small tasks

- Coping with sensory sensitivities

According to the World Federation of Occupational Therapists, "the primary goal of occupational therapy is to enable people to participate in the activities of everyday life." Specific activities will be based on your child's daily life and in what areas she is having difficulties. For example, if your child is having a hard time holding pencils or crayons or picking up small items, her occupational therapy exercises might include squeezing different size balls.

Social Skills Training

Social skills training is often done by different types of professionals and is often incorporated into various types of therapy. Your child might work with a speech language pathologist, a school guidance counselor, or a psychologist, who all teach social skills. These types of professionals work to improve simple social skills, such as making eye contact, the use of more abstract and social language, and more complex relationship skills. If your child is seeing several different professionals, it is very important that they coordinate their work so your child isn't confused by different styles or instructions about how to build more complex and appropriate social skills.

> **Aspie Advice**
>
> Social skills groups—often offered in treatment centers, through psychologists, or in school—give Aspies a chance to learn from one another in a safe environment. As your child matures and her social requirements change, you can reassess the group dynamics each year to make sure it still meets her needs. For example, are the group members the same age as her? Is she still learning new skills? Is the group evolving as skills are mastered?

Social skills are taught individually or in a group. Talk with your doctor, speech pathologist, psychologist, or school guidance office to find out whether a group for Aspies exists in your area. Group social programs mimic social situations and help Aspies learn to interact with one another in a safe, secure environment. Some groups go on field trips to help members practice social skills outside of the group as well while still being supportive of each other.

Applied Behavior Analysis

Applied Behavior Analysis (ABA) is used to reduce or minimize inappropriate behaviors or to build on daily living skills and communication skills. It uses the concept of positive reinforcement for desired behaviors and no reaction for undesired behaviors. Behavior therapists observe your child at home, in school, or wherever you are seeing problem behaviors. The therapist creates a plan of action to target specific areas. The process of formally developing a plan is called a Functional Behavioral Assessment or FBA, which can sometimes be provided through the public schools under Federal Laws like the Individuals with Disabilities Education Act, often simply referred to by educators as "IDEA."

Typical sessions are two to three hours long, with structured time focusing on a task or behavior, followed by breaks with free time. Behavior trainers use free play time to practice and reinforce skills in more natural circumstances. Sessions normally take place in your home, or the trainer can work with your child in different locations to help build skills in a variety of locations. Because an ABA program is customized to fit individual needs, each program looks different.

Assistive Technology

Assistive technology is any item, product, or piece of equipment that is used to help someone with a disability. These can be bought for a specific purpose or can be items purchased off the shelf and modified according to your child's needs. Assistive technology is as simple as photos to help your child remember chores to be completed or speech recognition software to help if your child is having a hard time writing.

Because many children with AS are visual learners, *visual representation systems* are often used. Some examples include:

- Pictures, photographs, or drawings combined with a schedule or calendar

- Social stories or scripts to help learn social rules

- Lists of chores

- Index cards with written reminders

- Written steps to aid in following directions

- Using pictures to aid in communication if your child has a hard time explaining what they want or need

Definition

Visual representation systems use objects, photographs, drawings, or written words to enhance the spoken word.

Visual representation systems are sometimes low-tech and created from items frequently found in your home or in the classroom. White boards to list the daily schedule or three-ring binders to keep steps for household chores help your child develop a sense of independence. More technologically advanced aids include using a video camera to record your child in social situations to teach inappropriate and appropriate social behaviors. Computers help in developing fine motor skills.

Another area in which assistive technology is widely used for adolescents with AS is in generating written material. The two main alternatives to putting a pen to paper are keyboarding and speech-to-text software for the computer. Many adolescents with Asperger's have difficulty communicating beyond merely handwriting problems. Aspies sometimes have difficulty getting ideas out onto paper with a pen or pencil. Sometimes using a keyboard can increase written work by several grade levels without any other intervention.

Medication

No medication can help directly with symptoms of AS. In Chapter 4, we explained related conditions, such as anxiety disorders, depression, and seizures. If your child is taking medication, it is probably to help with one or more of these conditions. Some medications your child may be taking include the following:

- Stimulant medications to help with symptoms of ADHD

- Antidepressants to help with anxiety or depression

- Anti-seizure medications

It is a good idea to keep a list of all the medications your child is taking and to research the possible side effects and drug interactions. Make sure every doctor has a copy of the list, and whenever a new medication is prescribed, talk about the side effects and possible interactions with other medications. Also, you should receive a "patient insert" each time you fill a prescription. Read this information carefully so you know what types of side effects to expect.

Your pharmacist is also a great source of information on both side effects and drug interactions. Using the same pharmacy to fill all of your child's prescriptions helps make sure dangerous interactions are avoided. Be sure to ask your pharmacist if there are any foods or drinks that should be avoided while taking certain medications and whether the medication should be taken with or without food.

Alternative Treatments

It is heartbreaking for you as a parent to watch your child struggle with symptoms of AS, and you may be tempted to search out new and alternative approaches. Some companies selling supplements advertise their products as a natural remedy to relieve AS symptoms or "cure" it. Some may give examples of how, after using their products, children no longer fit the criteria for AS, or by feeding your child a strict diet, you can make symptoms disappear. Unfortunately, these companies are willing to make money on your desperation. No cure exists for AS, and the time and effort put into trying different alternative treatments might be better spent helping your child to develop her individual strengths. Medical science proves that intensive treatments, such as those we discussed in this chapter, are the best approach to helping your child.

Researching Alternative Treatments

When looking into alternative treatments, do your research. Be aware that many companies are willing to sell you products or "new" therapies through misleading advertising. Ask for information on potential risks of any new treatment and know exactly what symptoms it is meant to help. Request information to back up claims of effectiveness and look for scientifically sound and well-documented data.

> **The Doctor's Take**
>
> You may hear about an alternative treatment called *chelation therapy.* Research does not indicate that it helps with AS, and it can result in death. In 2005, a boy in Pennsylvania received his third chelation therapy session at his doctor's office, went into cardiac arrest, and died. The FDA has approved chelation only for acute heavy-metal poisoning, and many state medical boards have advised their state's licensed physicians not to perform this treatment for autism spectrum disorders (ASDs).

Sometimes treatments can be harmful by themselves, but they can also interact with each other and either produce unexpected problems or minimize the benefits of a therapy that has already proven to help your child. Before beginning a new treatment program, ask for referrals. Talk with other parents about their experiences. If you belong to a support group or know other parents with children with AS, talk with them as well. Personal recommendations from others who have used a product or service rather than those supplied by the therapist or company are much more reliable. You should also speak with your doctor about any new treatment to make sure it won't interfere with therapies your child is already receiving.

Warnings About Supplements

If your child is a picky eater, you might be concerned about whether your child is getting enough nutrition and want to add supplements or vitamins. A number of companies sell supplements claiming to help reduce symptoms of AS. These supplements often contain calcium, fish oil, vitamin B_6, dimethylglycine (DMG), or L-carnosine. It is tempting to try these products; you don't need a prescription, and you can pick them up at your local drug store or supermarket. They are touted as "natural," and it is easy to believe that anything natural is beneficial.

But natural does not necessarily mean safe. Supplements are not regulated by the U.S. Food and Drug Administration (FDA). When you purchase a supplement, you don't receive a patient insert like you do with prescription medication that lists the possible side effects and interactions with other medications. Some supplements contain fillers that may or may not be natural and can be harmful in some cases. Lack of regulation can also result in wild variations in the actual amount of the active chemical in "natural" products so you can't rely on precisely what you are giving your child. Before giving your child any supplements, research possible side effects and talk to your doctor about whether they may cause interactions with other medications your child is taking.

Essential Takeaways

- The best treatment for AS is a combination of different therapies that target your child's unique symptoms.
- Your child's treatment team consists of several different types of medical professionals who must routinely communicate with one another.
- Occupational therapists help your child with daily living skills such as self-care, completing chores, and improving fine motor skills.
- Social skills therapy is often an essential for Aspies and speech language pathologists, counselors, psychologists, and social workers may be available to help with this therapy.
- It can be tempting to try supplements and alternative therapies, but it is important to talk to your child's doctor before beginning any new treatments.

Behaviors

Asperger's syndrome is not a behavioral disorder; however, there are a number of behaviors common in children with AS. In Part 2, we provide an overview of some of the main behaviors and thought processes: meltdowns, repetitive behaviors, literal or logical thinking, and perfectionism.

One of the major concerns of many parents is the tantrums or meltdowns that frequently happen. We explain the difference, giving you, as parents, an understanding of what may be behind the meltdown and offering suggestions on how to cope and reduce your child's meltdowns, including managing meltdowns in public places.

As with all behaviors, symptoms of AS change as your child matures. Meltdowns, while mostly physical in the early years, may be more verbal during the teen years; other symptoms such as rigid thinking may remain constant but need to be addressed differently depending on whether your child is a toddler or a teen. We address how behaviors and thought processes change and give tips on helping your child from his early years through early adulthood.

chapter 6

Common Behaviors and Thought Processes

Steps to take when your child has a meltdown

Dealing with the difficulty of rituals

Understanding idioms and figures of speech

How perfectionism provides a sense of security

Tanya knew it was a bad idea to stop at the grocery store on her way home from work. She had just picked up her son, Todd, from day care, and he seemed agitated. As soon as they got into the car, he said, "Did you see Max's cat?" He repeated this line from his favorite cartoon several times, which he often did when feeling stressed. But they were out of milk at home, and she knew Todd would want milk in his cereal the next morning. She decided it wouldn't be too bad to quickly run in the store and pick up milk.

She told Todd they were stopping at the store and explained they were just getting milk and then leaving. She told him what aisle the milk was in. But when they were in the store, Todd wanted the chocolate cookies he always ate, which were on the other side of the store.

When Tanya said "No, just milk," Todd became angry. He started yelling, screaming, pulling away from his mother, and running to the cookie aisle. Tanya could feel the stares, heard the unspoken words, and sensed the judgments about her poor parenting skills. She took a deep breath and walked calmly (even though she didn't feel calm) toward her son. Another day, another meltdown.

Tantrums and Meltdowns

Some confusion exists regarding the terms "tantrums" and "meltdowns" for parents of Aspies. Some believe that a meltdown is simply an overblown tantrum, and others believe each has distinct characteristics. The Merriam-Webster dictionary defines a tantrum as "a sudden fit of temper" and a meltdown as "a breakdown of self-control."

> **The Doctor's Take**
>
> Aspies are frequently immature emotionally, sometimes by several years. Keep both your child's chronological age and emotional maturity in mind when planning outings and social interactions.

Both can include yelling and screaming but may occur for different reasons. A tantrum normally happens because a child wants attention, freedom to do something, or a specific item. In other words, tantrums are a method to achieve a specific goal. During a tantrum your child might quickly look at you, just to check and see whether you are watching.

A meltdown, on the other hand, often happens as a result of stress overload. If your child is having a meltdown, chances are he doesn't care if you are watching. His actions are a way to release the anxiety and tension he is feeling. It sometimes seems as if the meltdown has its own power and won't stop until your child has expended all his energy or is removed from the situation.

Handling a Tantrum

For children without Asperger's syndrome (AS), temper tantrums normally occur between the ages of 1 and 4 and then disappear or become less and less frequent. While meltdowns are usually associated with AS, Aspies can have tantrums as well. Most parenting experts agree the best way to handle a temper tantrum is to not give in to your child's demands and to ignore his antics. After the temper tantrum is over, praise him for behaving correctly and move on to the next activity.

Dina wanted a cookie and when her mother said "no" she began crying. When that didn't work, Dina got louder and louder, screaming. Her mother ignored her, continuing to make dinner. When Dina finally realized she wasn't going to get a cookie, no matter how loudly she yelled, she started playing with the cat. Dina's mother commented on how well Dina was behaving. The tantrum was forgotten.

Meltdowns Are Communication

Meltdowns are not quite so easy. A meltdown may be triggered by not getting a cookie or a toy, but this is probably the "straw that broke the camel's back" rather than being the sole reason. A child with AS has meltdowns for multiple reasons and factors. Some common scenarios can be:

- Frustration or confusion when he doesn't understand others' behaviors
- Stress from unexpected changes in routine
- Feeling inadequate in sports or play because of a lack of muscle strength
- Wanting and needing social interaction but not knowing how to make friends
- Inability to express desires and feelings
- Sensory overstimulation
- When rushed, hurried, or in response to your stress

Because everyone reacts to stress differently, your child's meltdown doesn't necessarily look the same as other children's emotional outbursts. Some children become angry; others withdraw; some blame other children; some become aggressive. Aspies can lack the ability to regulate their emotions, so what may make a neurotypical child upset can send your child into a rage.

A meltdown is a release of negative feelings, and after it is over, your child feels better. This sense of relief can be a negative reinforcement to the behavior, giving your child the wrong idea that meltdowns are a good way to react to a high level of stress.

The Doctor's Take	How you deal with a meltdown is more important than trying to avoid it. You may not always be able to see the situation objectively. Talk to friends and relatives who have witnessed a meltdown and take notes on what events preceded it. Reviewing these notes can reveal patterns and provide ideas to prevent future episodes. The best long-term solution is to explore and develop appropriate alternative coping mechanisms for stress.

You know your child best. You can probably spot the warning signs that a meltdown is coming most of the time. To best help prevent and cope with meltdowns, use the following strategies:

List the warning signs. Write a list of signs that your child is becoming stressed. This might be agitation, more rigid thinking, flapping hands, or other repetitive behaviors. Starting when your child is around 9 or 10 years old, share this list with your child so he can be aware of the warning signs.

Provide alternate behaviors. Write down a list of actions your child can do to help head off a meltdown, such as going to another room or quiet area to calm down, listening to music, taking a soothing bath, asking for a massage, or interacting with his special interest. You can also include physical activities to help release excess anxiety such as using his video game exercise program, going outside for a walk, or going to the playground. Sometimes, creative destruction can be used—for example, smashing aluminum cans to take them to the recycle plant. When he feels stressed, he can choose from the list to help head off a meltdown.

Discuss the consequences. Explain to your child that he will need to apologize to anyone who is emotionally or physically hurt by his outburst.

Review the episode. After a meltdown, talk with your child about what he could have done and what he should do the next time this situation happens. You might want to use stories or scripts to help him have a specific plan for next time. Be careful, because he might begin to re-experience the emotional component of the meltdown if you get too detailed in your discussion of what was going on when it started.

When your child is having a meltdown, especially if it is in public, you probably feel embarrassed as well as frustrated. As soon as you see your child's warning signs, remove him from the situation. When in a store or restaurant, take him to the restroom, parking lot, or coatroom. Remain calm and, if able, ask him how he wants to solve the problem. Getting him involved in problem-solving can sometimes help distract him from the meltdown. Although it is hard to keep a positive attitude, getting angry or yelling at your child will only escalate the situation. Instead, take a deep breath, ignore the stares, and focus on what is important: your child.

If meltdowns are occurring frequently, watch carefully in the early stages of a meltdown for signs of seizures or have your child checked by a neurologist to be sure seizures are not contributing to outbursts. You can also meet with your child's behavior therapist to come up with some ideas on how to help your child manage his behavior when stressed. Here are some strategies and things for you to keep in mind:

- Sometimes you will have to wait out the meltdown. Remember that a meltdown doesn't last forever, and public meltdowns decrease as a child matures.

- Be creative in solving problems. Instead of never going out to eat, plan for an early dinner when the restaurants are not crowded or have dinner at home and go out for dessert after the dinner crowd has thinned out.

- Talk to school personnel about having a plan of action at school. Share your warning signs and come up with a few quiet places your child can go, such as the nurse's office or the library.

- Keep safety rules in mind during meltdowns; your child might become impulsive or irrational during the meltdown.

- Meltdowns are a form of communication; take a few minutes to try to figure out what your child is trying to tell you.

- Remember you have survived meltdowns before, and you will survive this one, too.

Above all, remember that meltdowns are hard on your child, too. He is probably mentally, physically, and emotionally exhausted when the meltdown is finished. Give him time to recover before going over rules or explaining what he could have done differently. Lectures are typically ineffective, but practicing what to do as an alternative can help your child choose new behaviors over old behaviors.

Coaches have known for centuries that you start practicing new skills under the lowest stress possible. As the person becomes more adept with the new skill, you gradually increase the stress under which they practice the skill to more closely approximate the real world. That's why football coaches start with shirts and pads, move to practice scrimmages, then regular games, and finally playoffs and championship games last. Try the same approach with your child for their stress-relieving skills.

Repetitive Behaviors and Rituals

One of the possible characteristics of AS is the presence of repetitive behaviors such as rocking back and forth, running fingers across a piece of cloth, wiggling toes, biting nails, or hand flapping. Although not all people with AS display these behaviors, they are fairly common. These movements may be your child's way of calming down or a way to provide stimulation when understimulated. As with Todd in the previous section, it can also be words or phrases repeated over and over. Sometimes these movements or words must be repeated a certain number of times and can become a part of your child's daily routine. They can be extremely obvious or subtle, so that most people would not even notice the behavior.

You may worry about repetitive behaviors looking like tics, as in *Tourette's syndrome,* but there are differences. Tourette's syndrome movements usually begin around the age of 6 or 7 years old, while repetitive behaviors in AS can begin before a child is 2 years old. In AS, these movements are often a reaction to excitement or stress; in Tourette's syndrome, stress can increase the tics, but they are not limited to stressful situations.

Definition

Tourette's syndrome is a neuropsychiatric disorder characterized by repetitive and involuntary movements and vocal behaviors called tics. Tics can be "simple," such as eye blinking, shoulder shrugging, throat clearing, or saying a word. Complex tics are patterns of movement that include several muscle groups such as jumping or bending and often involve repeating phrases. Children with mild Tourette's syndrome may not require any treatment, but more severe cases might require medication.

Repetitive behaviors can also be compulsions or rituals. Your child might line up toys in a certain way, going back several times to make sure they are lined up correctly or having to put his things away in a certain order before going to bed. He may need to watch the same show at the same time each day, read the same story before bed, or count the same items each day. Repetitive behaviors are as varied and unique as each child.

Many people indicate that rituals are one of the most difficult aspects of AS, because your child may be totally inflexible in performing routines. When routines are interrupted, frustration and meltdowns can occur. Your family's daily schedule may need to take your child's routines into account. Outings can throw your child into despair if he is not home to complete the ritual. Other children may get annoyed or frustrated that they must plan their day around these rituals.

Often planning minor disruptions when you know you will have the time, energy, and resources to handle them can be a good way of helping your child deal with real-world interruptions in his rituals when they do happen. This sort of long-term planning helps to minimize the negative impact that such rigidity has on the Aspie and his family.

Aspie Advice

Be creative in finding solutions for interrupted or delayed rituals. One family was going to a family wedding. Their son, Rudy, couldn't fall asleep until he knew his cars were "properly" lined up under this bed. His parents allowed Rudy to line up the cars in the trunk of their car. Rudy knew the cars were close by and was able to fall asleep on the way home, saving his family a difficult ride home.

Obsessive compulsive disorder (OCD), an anxiety disorder, includes strict rituals or repetitive behaviors, but as with tantrums and meltdowns, the reasons behind the behaviors are different. In children with AS, the behaviors and rituals provide a sameness and sense of order. In children with

OCD, rituals and behaviors are a way to reduce anxiety and fear. In OCD, thoughts and behaviors are intrusive and unwanted, but Aspies are not bothered by their thoughts and do not find them invasive or bothersome. It is possible for a child to be diagnosed with both AS and OCD, but this combination is often inappropriate because rituals are often calming for an Aspie but are distressing for someone with OCD. Additionally, medications intended for OCD, and often very effective for traditional OCD cases, are less likely to be effective for people with AS.

- Use repetitive actions and rituals to help calm your child during times of excitement or agitation.

- Share certain rituals (those that won't be the cause of teasing, such as interacting with a toy that is below his age level) with your child's teacher to give her a way to help your child remain calm during school.

- As your child gets older, teach him what rituals should not be completed out of the house, including those that might cause other children to tease him.

A Literal Way of Thinking

Your child probably thinks in concrete, literal terms. He believes that people mean what they say and say what they mean. He has trouble with *idioms,* figures of speech, and may take words exactly as they are, not paying attention to tone of voice or inflections that help give meaning. He may not like books or cartoons in which animals talk or wear clothes because it doesn't make sense to him; he may prefer realistic stories, ones about people and real-life situations.

definition

An **idiom** is an expression of speech in which the meaning cannot be derived by using context clues and is often used by a particular group of people. For example, teenagers might use the idiom "chill out" to mean relax.

We use different figures of speech every day and because they have become ingrained in our speech, we don't realize how they sound to our children.

Consider the following scenario. Debra and her family were having dinner and 8-year-old Jonas was telling a story about something that had happened in school. Debra said, "You're pulling my leg." Jonas looked very confused, "No, Mommy, I'm not pulling your leg, don't you see me sitting here eating dinner?" Jonas didn't understand it was a figure of speech; he thought his mother really thought he was under the table pulling on her leg.

Keep a notebook with figures of speech and what they mean. Go over them with your child and add more as he comes into contact with others. The following are some examples of idioms and figures of speech that might confuse him. As you read them, imagine what he would think if he heard them.

- Cat got your tongue
- Keep your eye on the ball
- Run to the store
- Hop on the bus
- A little bird told me
- I've changed my mind
- Break a leg
- Costs an arm and a leg
- At the drop of a hat
- Tickled pink or feeling blue
- Caught with his pants down
- He was on fire
- Feeling under the weather

As he reaches the teen years, keep up with popular phrases and add them to your book so he does not feel so out of place when classmates use phrases he does not understand—for example, "chill out" and "hang out."

Window Shopping

MISC.

One family was shopping in a home improvement store. After the parents had picked up the items they needed, they continued browsing. Joey, their 12-year-old Aspie, asked his parents what they were looking for, and the father replied, "We're window shopping." Joey walked away and started down toward the other end of the store. When his father asked him where he was going, he replied, "The windows are down this way."

When speaking with your child, it's helpful to keep in mind these literal interpretations. Try to talk to him in concrete terms. Asking your child "Are you ready to go?" may get you a "Yes" without him moving from where he is. Instead, state, "We are leaving now, please come along."

People on the autism spectrum often have difficulty with generalizing from the situation in which they learn a skill to new or novel situations in which the same skill or behavior is also appropriate. When you tell your child what to do in a certain situation, he may assume the rule is only for that situation and can't apply the information to similar situations. For example, if your son burps at the kitchen table and you say, "It is not polite to burp at the table," you may be embarrassed later when he stands up at a friend's house, steps back from the table, and loudly burps. You need to explain when rules apply to more than one place or situation.

Two additional rules to keep in mind:

- Teach your child to ask "Are you joking?" or "I am confused, can you explain that?" when they don't understand.

- Avoid using general pronouns such as them, those, and their. Instead use the specific words.

Anything Less Than Perfect Is Unacceptable

A perfectionist strives to be perfect; anything less is unacceptable. Aspies are often motivated more by avoiding errors and mistakes than they are by being "right." This often leads to both the aforementioned obsessive behaviors and to rigid or perfectionist behaviors.

Achieving Perfection

Your child may require a sense of order around him to feel safe and secure. This need for order requires everything to be right. He doesn't like mistakes in him or those around him. For example, Aspies frequently correct others when speaking. In their mind, the other person appreciates the corrections, because why would someone not want correct information? Teachers, adult relatives, or even an acquaintance you meet in the grocery store don't understand; instead, they think your child is rude, impertinent, and arrogant.

> **The doctor's Take**
>
> Perfectionism is more apparent during transitions, such as entering middle school or high school or moving to a new neighborhood. Because of the stress generated by not knowing what is expected of him in the new environment, your child might have a strong desire to do everything exactly right and be afraid of making mistakes.

Communication often doesn't come easy for an Aspie, but when a conversation involves something he knows about, your child feels comfortable speaking up. He is the expert and, when corrected, may have a hard time accepting it. He may only accept the word of someone else he views as an "expert" on the topic. Other children may see him as a "know it all" and avoid being with him, or worse, ridicule him in front of peers.

Perfectionism goes beyond conversation. Your child may painstakingly spend hours completing a homework assignment, making sure every letter is formed correctly; every answer right. He may refuse to hand in assignments that are not perfect. For you, trying to help with homework can be a nightmare. If it is not explained exactly like the teacher explained it, you are wrong. If you don't complete the problem with exactly the same steps as he was shown in school, he gets upset. Taking tests is also hard. Your child prefers to have the right answer, no matter how long it takes. Timed tests are difficult to finish because he needs to erase and rewrite answers over and over.

Avoiding Errors

Besides needing order, another reason for perfectionism is the fear of making a mistake. Your child can go to great lengths to avoid errors because he is afraid of failing. He needs to be perfect because he thinks that is the way to fit in and be accepted socially. Your child may not understand that other people make mistakes. Because he doesn't read behind words and actions, he assumes that everyone else can do whatever it is correctly, the first time. He assumes he is the only person that doesn't "get it." He may dread being ridiculed by classmates for mistakes. One of the biggest insults to an Aspie is calling them "stupid." This is because he sees errors as a serious problem and thinks people who make repeated errors are "stupid."

As a parent, you can lead by example, let your child know when you have made a mistake, and talk through it out loud. Let him know that throughout history mistakes have led to great discoveries, inventions, and even chocolate chip cookies:

- Ruth Wakefield was making chocolate cookies to serve to the guests at Toll House Inn and realized she didn't have any baker's chocolate. Instead, she broke up pieces of sweetened chocolate and put them in the cookies, expecting the cookies to become chocolate while they baked. Instead she invented the most popular kind of cookie today.

- Ice cream cones were created when an ice cream vendor at the World's Fair in 1904 ran out of dishes for serving his ice cream. The vendor next to him was selling a thin Persian waffle. He rolled up a waffle, topped it with the ice cream, and invented the ice cream cone.

- Post-It Notes were invented from a failed experiment. A man named Spencer Silver worked for 3M Company and was trying to invent a strong glue. Instead the glue was weak, and he didn't know what to do with it. Years later, a scientist he had worked with was frustrated with markers always falling out of his hymnal at church and used the weak glue to hold them in place without ripping the pages. The glue was then used to create Post-It Notes.

Aspie Advice   Always praise efforts instead of focusing on the end result. Children who are perfectionists are afraid of getting a bad grade or not reaching the end goal. Reassure your child that it is the effort that counts; a child who works hard and receives a "C" in class is not a failure. One of the best ways to say this is "You can always be proud of yourself if you did your best."

These stories show how mistakes aren't always bad and that "failures" sometimes lead to successes. Explain to your child that mistakes are how we learn. Help your child to see that the goal of homework, schoolwork, and other activities is to learn, not necessarily to get every question right. Share your own stories of how you have made mistakes in the past and how some of those have helped you to learn and grow.

Essential Takeaways

- Meltdowns and tantrums are similar but occur for different reasons.
- Repetitive behaviors and rituals help Aspies to relax and calm down when feeling stressed.
- Aspies have logical, linear thought processes. Talking to Aspies in specific, concrete ways helps them to process information.
- Perfectionism can come from a fear of making a mistake.

chapter 7

How Behaviors Change with Age

Understanding patterns of behavior in toddlers

Setting foundation rules for young children

Creating behavioral systems in your household

Changes in preteen years

Fostering independence in a teen with AS

Asperger's syndrome (AS) is a lifelong condition. No cure magically takes away symptoms or makes your child "normal," but as she grows, behaviors change. In the early years your child may throw herself on the floor, arms and legs flailing, and in the teenage years tantrums are often more verbal than physical. As a parent, you also change how you deal with difficult behaviors as your child changes. In this chapter, we explain how behaviors change in different stages of development and how parents can adapt to these changes.

Infant and Toddler Years

AS is usually diagnosed at around 11 years old in the United States but can be diagnosed as early as 3 to 4 years old. Many parents report seeing signs of AS from the time their children are very young or at least knowing there was something "different" about their children. Newborns, although they may be fussy and irritable during times of high stimulation or when around strangers, don't really have "behavioral" problems. Refer to Chapter 2 for a list of some of the early warning signs of AS.

Tantrums and meltdowns start to appear during the toddler years. Children without AS learn to communicate their wants, needs, and feelings using both words and actions. As they continue to learn new words and ways to communicate, tantrums decrease. Even though Aspies have a large vocabulary and are verbal, it is hard for them to explain feelings, especially when overwhelmed.

The Doctor's Take	It is easy to be hard on yourself and judge your parenting skills based on how many meltdowns your child has each day or week. By doing that, you will likely end up feeling like a failure if your child has a bad day. Instead, focus on your response to the meltdowns and on progress.

Sensory issues are a common reason for meltdowns during the toddler years. Usually, at this age, children have not yet been diagnosed with AS, and parents don't understand what is going on.

Joshua was 3 years old. His mother, Jenna, still dressed him each morning because, if she left it to him, he would go without clothes. Getting him dressed was a major battle, but putting on socks and shoes often ended up in a meltdown. The seams in the socks had to be just right. Jenna started out patiently, putting on the socks, straightening out the seams, and slowly putting on the shoes to make sure the seams didn't move. Some mornings Jenna would go through this process several times, with Joshua getting more and more frustrated each time. Some mornings he would cry and fuss, and other mornings he would take off his shoes, throw them across the room, and refuse to put them back on.

Jenna didn't understand what was going on. She had older children, and none had acted like this. Putting on shoes and socks was a pretty simple task, and she had no idea why it was so hard with Joshua. She tried shoes without socks, but he didn't like the feel of them and would still take his shoes off. Jenna looked forward to summer, when he could wear sandals and, although she was embarrassed to admit it, sometimes allowed him to wear the sandals in the middle of winter, ignoring the stares of other parents and imagining they all thought she was a terrible parent.

As a parent, learning about the patterns behind meltdowns helps you cope with and manage the behaviors. It might be helpful for you to keep a diary of your child's tantrums and meltdowns. Pay attention to when this behavior occurs most often and when it is least likely to occur. For example, does your child have tantrums at a certain time of day? Are his meltdowns a "last straw," showing your child can tolerate a certain amount of frustration? Do meltdowns happen when routines are changed? Write down what happens before a meltdown. This information helps you to look for patterns. The more detail your log contains, the easier it will be to see patterns and find triggers to the meltdowns when you sit down and review them.

During the toddler years, you may begin to see repetitive movements. During times of stress, your child may flap his hands, rock back and forth, or spin around. Being aware of the movements he makes when agitated helps you monitor and take steps to reduce further stress. Your child may also use these types of movements to help calm down.

Aspie Advice

Know the signs of a meltdown. Although each child is different, you might see physical signs such as a loss of coordination, sweating, hyperventilation, paleness, or flushing of the face, or your child might complain of stomachaches. Some Aspies begin to retreat into a favorite hobby by quoting sayings or passages or by beginning a "mini-lecture" on the topic out of the blue.

During this stage of development, you should create ground rules for behavior, such as no hitting or biting, so your child knows what is expected of him. You should also create daily routines so he knows what to expect. If your log of behaviors showed meltdowns occurring at a certain time each day, set up some "downtime" in the routine shortly before he normally gets overwhelmed. This downtime could be watching a video, playing a computer game, or spending quiet time in his room. Remember, what is relaxing for one person is not necessarily for another, so select downtime based on what he finds relaxing. Being proactive and consistent will help your toddler begin to develop self-control.

Ages 4 to 7 Years

At this age range, children—especially those who have not yet been diagnosed—appear to outsiders to be spoiled. Aspies seem to ignore others, are absorbed in their own little worlds, and no matter how parents try, they can be impossible to reason with. While your friends' children have started to outgrow tantrums, yours hasn't. The tantrums continue at home and in public. The ones in public are the worst. You try to be calm, but you can feel the stares of other people. You know they think you are the worst parent who walked the earth. Some well-meaning onlookers even try to give you advice, "You know when you give in to a tantrum it only makes it worse" or "You should try disciplining him; that would make him stop." The embarrassment makes you want to stay home. At least if there is a meltdown, it is in the privacy of your own living room, and you can handle it as you see best, without the judgment of those around you.

Staying home isn't the answer. Staying home punishes your entire family because your child has AS. It makes you feel like an outcast. Other children in the family end up resentful, because they don't understand why they should never be able to go out to dinner or go shopping at the mall. And your child doesn't learn how to navigate the outside world, which means there is little chance that the problem behaviors will go away.

Some parents type up small cards with information on AS. One parent wrote, "My child has Asperger's syndrome. Meltdowns are common in children with AS and often happen in times of overexcitement or over-stimulation. I understand and appreciate your concern. The best thing you can do is to allow me time and space to help my child regain his sense of safety and security." When her child had a meltdown in public, she handed out the cards to those closest to her. This allowed her to respond to those around her without engaging in a verbal discussion that would add to her stress. Most onlookers responded by quietly moving away. Refer to the previous chapter for other ways you can handle tantrums and meltdowns in public.

Fears Related to AS Symptoms

Misc.

One report, "The Fears, Phobias and Anxieties of Children with Autism Spectrum Disorders and Down Syndrome" by David W. Evans and others, showed that children with an autism spectrum disorder were more likely to have situational fears but had less fears of harm and injury than other children. Their fears were directly related to the symptoms of ASD.

Your child may have certain phobias and fears. He may be afraid of the vacuum cleaner or have a fear of water. At times, you may feel that you are running your household according to his fears. For example, you can only vacuum when he is away from the house, or you spend an hour or two in the evening getting your child clean because he doesn't want to get wet.

During this stage, you may also begin to see rigid behaviors and difficulty transitioning. Your child may become agitated when his routine is changed, at some times refusing to participate in other activities until after he has completed the first task. He may need things done in a certain way. For example, Jeff would not eat dinner unless he had the dish and cup with his favorite cartoon character on it. On nights when the dish was in the dishwasher or not yet washed from lunch, his parents tried to reason with him, explaining that all dishes were the same, but Jeff would sit at the table not eating anything if there was a different plate in front of him. They ended up buying a few plates and making sure there was always a clean plate at mealtime. Your child probably feels most comfortable when the same routine is followed every day. He wants to watch the same video, at the same time every day. He needs to go through the same ritual each night before going to bed. When the routine is changed, even a little, he reacts with anger and frustration.

Aspie Advice

When teaching your child a new skill, present the different ways it can be completed to help develop flexible thinking and ask others to participate, too. For example, when giving your child a paper to draw on, show him it is okay to draw when the paper is placed in a landscape position or a portrait position. This helps him accept doing things in more than one way and with more than one person.

Perfectionism can start appearing around this age. Your child might get frustrated if he can't do something the way he thinks it should be done. This can show up in two main ways: he might give up, or he won't bother to try. At this age, it is sometimes hard to tell the difference between rigidity and perfectionism, because both can cause tempers to flare if something isn't done the "right" way either by the Aspie or by others.

In the toddler years, it is important to set down some foundation rules for behavior. Between ages 4 and 7, it is time to set up a system for your household:

- Always try to see what the behavior is trying to tell you. All behavior is a form of communication. Look past the behavior to see the meaning before reacting.

- Be consistent in your approaches and stay positive. When your child is having a meltdown, it can be hard to be positive. If you have followed the preceding advice and understand he is simply communicating with you, it will be easier.

- Set rewards for desired behaviors. This can be as simple as praising your child when you see him behaving appropriately. When first starting a reward program, it is important to "catch" your child behaving as often as possible.

- Allow your child to make choices whenever possible. For example, let your child pick out what clothes to wear or offer several foods and let him choose which one he wants. This helps him to feel he has some control over his life.

- Help your child experience success. Work with your child to create goals, such as dressing himself. Make sure the goals are doable so your child can achieve them and feel good. Remember the two measures of success—did he try his best, and did he do better than the last time?

- Do not fall into the trap of becoming rigid yourself in reaction to your child's challenges. This can be seductive because it solves and prevents problems short-term, but this rigidity will create more intense rigidity from him in the long term.

Ages 8 to 11

At this age range, you may find that you have settled into a routine, and the tantrums and meltdowns have decreased. Your child knows what to expect and has learned ways to communicate his needs. Family life is somewhat peaceful with an occasional meltdown when your child is overwhelmed. For other families, this age is tough. Your child may have a hard time fitting in at school and teasing from the other students might make every day miserable. His inability to regulate his emotions causes him to overreact, situations are blown out of proportion, and he flies into a rage over what you see as small problems.

In addition to using the advice in the previous section, work with your child on creating a conflict resolution chart. List different situations and emotions and give your child different choices of behaviors he can choose from. For example:

> *Situation:* Being teased by a classmate makes you mad.

> *You can:* Walk away and find a different activity, ask the classmate to stop, ignore the classmate, or talk to the teacher about what is going on.

By thinking up different situations and offering your child a choice of behaviors, you make him feel more in control and help prepare him for new situations.

When your child was younger, he may not have been interested in interacting with other children. He may have been content being by himself. At this age, he may start being aware of his differences but doesn't understand what the other children are talking about or why they act in certain ways. He says things at the wrong time and talks too much about his interests. His classmates reject his attempts to join conversations. He wants friends and wants to be included, but day after day he isn't. Because he can't always explain how he is feeling, his frustration comes out in other ways, frequently as anger or meltdowns.

Aspies are more emotionally immature than their peers, sometimes by as much as three to four years at this age. If your child is more interested in playing with children younger than him, he could be choosing friends who are at the same level of maturity. Helping him increase his social sophistication gradually can make him more comfortable with peers his own age.

As a parent, it is important that you appreciate every achievement your child makes, no matter how small. It could be tying his shoes by himself, getting along with a classmate, or making it through dinner without monopolizing the conversation. When you live with someone day in and day out, it is sometimes hard to see the changes. Take the time to look for any improvement and praise your child for each one. Many times we look at our children based on where we think they should be developmentally, academically, and socially. To help your child succeed, look at where he is today and base achievements on that place instead.

During this stage, your child should be able to be included in problem solving. He should be able to understand why meltdowns, especially in public, are not appropriate behaviors and know what types of behaviors are more acceptable. It is important for him to know that it is okay to feel angry or frustrated, but it is not okay to hit. Work together with your child to find solutions and to figure out what he could do when he is feeling stressed or overwhelmed. Listen to his suggestions and try to use them when creating your conflict resolution chart.

Preteen and Early Teen Years

The preteen and early teen years are a time of great transitions and changes, neither of which are easy for your child. Some parents find these years the most difficult. During this time, not only is your child's body beginning to change, but social relationships take on different dimensions. Relationships were previously based on activities and interests. If a classmate liked the same toy, your child had something to talk about; if they both were interested in cars or dolls, they could relate based on this. Now relationships are based on conversation, personalities, and sharing thoughts and ideas. In addition, language changes at this age from generally concrete to including more and more abstract language, which is typically the weakest language area for Aspies. For children with AS, literal thinking often creates misunderstandings.

Christy suddenly didn't want to go to school. In the morning she stayed in her room, and when her mother called her for school she refused to come out. Her mother was concerned that other students were teasing Christy and asked her if the other students were saying mean things. "No," Christy said, "I was playing with some of the girls at recess yesterday, and they were picking out boys to marry. Rhonda said I needed to marry Jim, and I don't want to marry him!" When Christy's mom explained that this was a game that girls play and that no one expected her to actually marry Jim, Christy felt a little better. She still didn't understand the game or why you would say you were going to marry someone when you didn't mean it, but she accepted that the other girls didn't expect her to marry Jim at recess that day and agreed to go to school.

The preteen and early teen years, for all children, are filled with demanding behavior, angry outbursts, and mood changes as they try to navigate a more mature world they don't understand yet. This isn't anything new to your child; he has been living in a world he doesn't understand all his life. But your child is now facing new and more confusing situations, and his peers are less consistent than in the past, which does not help him know how to behave in response. The constant pressure to keep up with classmates can have your child acting out both at home and in school. Meltdowns, even if they had slowed down over the past couple of years, can start back up.

> **The Doctor's Take**
>
> When sending your child to her room to calm down, make sure you stress that this is not a punishment; that this time is to help her learn how to regulate her emotions.

Around this time you begin to wonder about discipline. You worry that if you punish your child, you are punishing him for having AS. At the same time, you don't want to ignore inappropriate behaviors. How can you distinguish between behaviors caused by AS and normal tween behavior? Your focus should be on acceptable/unacceptable behaviors instead of worrying what is causing the behavior. You may handle the behaviors differently, for example, if your child acts out because of AS, and you may need to allow extra time for him to calm down before talking about the inappropriate behavior and working on what could have been done differently.

In the previous section, we discussed setting up a conflict resolution chart. As your child matures, you should revise the chart, focusing on current situations he is facing. Besides listing actions to resolve differences, provide him with specific actions to take when he wants something.

Adolescence

The main symptoms of AS don't change as your child grows. Problems with social skills, literal thinking, and intense interests continue throughout his life. But there are differences in how these symptoms show up. For example, when your child was young, he may not have been interested in developing relationships with classmates and may have been content spending large blocks of time alone. As your child enters the teen years, he faces a whole new set of problems. Teachers have higher expectations, friendships change, and teens begin to explore romantic relationships.

While parents often find the preteen years the most difficult, Aspies find the teen years the most difficult. Other teens are not only discovering romantic relationships but are gaining independence from their parents, looking toward graduating from high school, and going away to college. Your child probably isn't ready for the same level of independence as his peers. Even though many teens with AS see a jump in maturity during the teen years, your child still needs help understanding the world around him. All teens resent their parents holding on, and teens with AS are no exception. Tantrums and meltdowns reappear. When he was little, meltdowns were physical events, but as teens, meltdowns become verbal confrontations.

| Aspie Advice | As with neurotypical teens, talking with parents is frequently a last resort. It is a good idea to find a trusted adult—maybe a teacher, a relative, or a family friend—for your teen to talk with. |

Typical teen behavior includes being moody, unpredictable, or uncommunicative, and all of these behaviors can be exacerbated (or heightened) in Aspies. Other teens are able to talk about the changes in their bodies, romantic relationships, and plans for their future, but social conversations are difficult for your child. He may not have any friends to share information with. If he does have friends, talking about emotions and feelings is hard. Because anxiety and depression are common in Aspies, look over the signs discussed in Chapter 4 and seek medical help if you think your teen may be depressed.

Passions can intensify at this time, sometimes because it is a way to relax and let go of the stresses of the day. As a parent, you may want to take the time to learn about your teen's interests to give you a way to continue connecting. Special interests will be discussed in detail in Chapter 8, but for now keep in mind that these interests can be used as a way to expand your teen's interest and as a general direction for career paths. There may be times, however, that you will need to limit the time your teen spends on his interest, bringing some balance to his life.

Focus on the positive. Use the strategies you have developed throughout your child's life. Sometimes the teen years seem like a whole different world, but understand how your child thinks and acts. Remember you have survived the younger years; you will survive the teen years. You are in a better position than parents of neurotypical teens who haven't lived with tantrums and meltdowns throughout the earlier years.

Young Adult Years

As high school ends, another phase—the young adult—begins. This stage can be more frightening for parents than the high school years. Should your child go to college? If so, should he stay at home and attend a local college, or is going away to college better? If your child isn't ready for college, what type of job is best? You might be confused and not know what is best for your child.

Many young adults with AS are academically ready for college but may not be prepared in other ways. The higher demands of college classes demand organization and time management. Being able to study, do laundry, clean his dorm room, and manage class schedules every day requires the ability to multitask. Your child needs to be able to manage money and finances. All of these responsibilities are new and scary.

Your child may not want to go to college. He might find academics overwhelming and be glad to leave school behind him. He might instead want to go to work. Whether heading off to college or looking for a job, your child probably still needs your help.

> **The Doctor's Take**
>
> Preparation for adulthood starts well before graduation. Give your Aspie more responsibility to help him become independent. Having responsibility also means having the chance of failing, dealing with the results of not doing something at all or not doing it correctly. If you allow your child to experience this early, while you're around to soften the consequences, he is much more likely to be ready to tackle the demands of being at college or holding down a "real" job later.

Young adults with AS are apt to reject any advice from their parents. They want independence and want to make their own decisions. You, being nervous about the future, want to hold on a little longer, afraid your child isn't ready to face the outside world alone. Conflict between you and your child often increases. If your child has been seeing a therapist, talk with her about whether she believes your child is ready to live independently. If so, she can help both you and your child make the transition from living at home to living either at college or in an apartment.

Remember that you need to create an adult life for your child based on his dreams. Throughout his life, you probably envisioned a certain future and had to adjust these based on your child's abilities to function on his own. Keep communication open so you know what your child wants and looks forward to. Work to help his dreams become a reality.

Essential Takeaways

- Sensory issues are one of the causes of meltdowns in toddlers.
- Your family frequently feels they are ruled by the fears and phobias of your child with AS.
- Creating a conflict resolution chart helps give your child choices for handling difficult situations.
- The preteen years are often a difficult time for parents of a child with AS.
- In the teen years, meltdowns change from physical to verbal.

Managing Obsessions

One of the hallmark signs of Asperger's syndrome (AS) is an intense, focused interest on a specific topic. Boys with AS may be preoccupied with topics revolving around transportation or science while girls may have an intense interest in animals or characters from books or movies. This interest often permeates every aspect of family life, from dinner table conversations to themes for the family vacation. In Part 3, we discuss why these interests are important to your child.

You may be concerned if your child's passion is inappropriate such as a fixation on weapons, pornography, or even on another person. We offer ideas for handling this situation and discuss times when parents need to limit access to special interests.

There are many ways you, as a parent, can use your child's special interest to help him learn about the world around him. We provide ways to use passions as motivation, as educational tools, to help him expand interests, to build social skills, and even to choose a career. Finally, we talk about how special interests change throughout your child's life, from the early years throughout early adulthood.

chapter 8

Special Interests

Special interests as a relaxation tool

Short-term versus long-term passions

Steps to take when special interests are inappropriate

Using passions as educational tools

Limiting access to special interests

Brian, at 11 years old, was fascinated with dinosaurs. His interest had started a few years ago and soon he knew an enormous amount of information about dinosaurs. He could name every dinosaur, when each roamed the Earth, what they ate, when each was discovered, and much more. Every morning he checked the television listings to see whether there was a show on television about dinosaurs. In his room there was a stack of books on dinosaurs he looked through every night before going to sleep. Many of the books were well beyond those written for his age, but he didn't mind, and actually those were the ones he looked through most often because the ones written for children only had basic information. He needed more.

Every morning when Brian arrived at school he went directly to his teacher and talked about dinosaurs, telling her what he had read the night before, even if it was the same litany he had told her many times before. Every day when he arrived home, he took out his dinosaur figures and disappeared into his room until it was time to do his homework. At dinner, he recited facts about dinosaurs.

Brian, like most children with Asperger's syndrome (AS), has fixated on a topic and spends a great deal of time reading, studying, and learning everything about it, and his interest often monopolizes his conversations. These special interests are sometimes compared to hobbies. Many children come home from school and spend time on hobbies, such as video games or baseball; many adults come home from work and spend time on their hobbies, such as puttering in the garden. Hobbies help us relax; they let us transition from work to home, putting the stresses of our day behind us. The special interests of children with AS do the same thing; the difference is in the intensity of the interest.

The Importance of Special Interests

It is hard to see how an obsession on a single, narrow focus benefits your child. As someone without AS, you know the value of a well-rounded life. You understand balance. You spend a portion of your day at work, another portion as a caregiver to your family, and a portion delving into your own interests. You can't imagine hour after hour, day after day focused in one area. But for Aspies, special interests are important for a number of reasons.

MISC.

What Interests Your Child?

Special interests can be about any topic. Some are unusual—for example, an interest in batteries, vacuum cleaners, or pots and pans. A few of the more common special interests include a specific animal, even those that are extinct today; transportation, such as trains or trucks; computer games; Japanese anime; or science fiction films.

Relaxation and Enjoyment

As we discussed in Chapter 4, many Aspies develop an anxiety disorder, and special interests help in defraying some of the daily stress your child feels. Just as working in the garden, knitting, or reading help you wind down from a hectic day, for a child with AS, gathering information or interacting with his special interest allows him time to let go of the stress of trying to communicate and live in a non-Asperger's world, even for a little while.

One of the myths about Aspies is they are not able to experience pleasure. Because of their difficulty expressing emotion and sharing emotion with others in their lives, it is mistakenly assumed they are not able to feel these emotions. But many individuals with AS report feeling pleasure and enjoyment when spending time interacting with their special interests and during other activities.

Order and Consistency

Many Aspies don't like surprises; they want their lives to be structured and ordered. This helps your child feel safe and secure in a world he doesn't understand and lets the chaos of the outside world slip away. Aspies set their own terms for interacting with interests, reading, researching on the internet, watching videos, acting out, drawing, or modeling behaviors. Many follow a set routine, waking up each morning and watching a video or looking through a book before beginning the day. Your child's day may be planned with breaks that allow him to spend time interacting with his interest.

> **The Doctor's Take**
>
> If you have to take away or change the time your child spends with his special interest, try to plan ahead. Explain the change in routine, why it is needed, and give an alternative time to pursue his interest. If possible, write down the new schedule and when the schedule is to return to normal. For more permanent changes, some children benefit from well-planned transitions to the new schedule or routine, while for others this preplanning increases their stress about the change. You know your child, and what approach works best varies from child to child, so use these suggestions to guide you in having a plan that is most likely to help with your child.

Although many parents of Aspies try to keep days consistent, changes are inevitable. Children grow up and have to go to school, weekends are different than weekdays, and summers are different than the school year. Each year brings changes to their lives and to those around them. As children grow up, expectations of what they do change. These constant changes are a source of frustration, and the special interest brings consistency; no matter what goes on around your child, the special interest is the same.

Intellectual Appearance

Another myth about Aspies is that they are not smart. This is not true and, in fact, cognitive delays would prevent a child from being diagnosed with AS. Individuals with AS usually have a normal IQ or above.

Because of their inability to read social cues or effectively communicate, Aspies may be seen as less intelligent, and gathering a large body of information on a specific topic helps them to show others they are not lacking in intelligence. Aspies might use a specific language or terminology based on a special interest. For example, an interest in insects would include words such as "arthropods" or "exoskeleton." Using this type of terminology reminds others that your child is not stupid.

Additionally, many Aspies are motivated more by a desire to avoid being wrong than by a great desire to be right, as we discussed in Chapter 6. For these Aspies, amassing a large body of information on one subject helps assure them that they will not be "wrong."

Conversation Confidence

Usually, Aspies are not very good at making conversation. They don't understand small talk and feel uncomfortable entering conversations that are already taking place. A high level of information on a topic gives your child something to talk about with other children and with adults. Being knowledgeable helps your child feel as if he has something to contribute to conversations. The plus side is that he has something to talk about; the minus side is that he only has one thing to talk about at any length.

An Escape

Living with Asperger's syndrome too often makes children feel isolated and alone, unaccepted by their peers, and possibly bullied or teased on a daily basis. Special interests often offer an alternative world, one in which your child is accepted for who he is. Drawing from the interest, your child may create a safe, secure place where he feels comfortable with his differences and where those differences don't matter. This is normally not harmful, as long as parents watch to make sure the line between make-believe and the real world does not become too blurry.

Because special interests are usually solitary activities, your child doesn't need, and may not want, anyone else involved. Some special interests give Aspies a group to interact with who share their passion for that area or topic. It is not unusual for bright Asperger's teens to interact with adults who are professionals in their area of interest. This can be as lofty as discussing very detailed issues around one specific fossil find with a university archeologist or as routine as attending a science fiction convention and interacting over the specifics of a particular movie or television show.

Sense of Identity

When you think about yourself and who you are, you may think of roles in your relationships, such as mother, sister, or daughter, or your job, such as teacher or pharmacist. You may describe yourself using personality traits, such as funny or serious. Many Aspies identify themselves with their interest. Based on the amount of research a child has done, he very likely is a small expert on the topic. It gives him a sense of identity and purpose.

> **Aspie Advice**
>
> Acceptance and appreciation of your child's passion can go a long way to help improve his self-image. For some, the special interest doesn't make sense to parents or classmates. For example, a young child may have a burning desire to learn about washing machines or drain covers. But as the child's expertise grows, he gains respect for his extensive knowledge. Embracing a fascination, even when it doesn't make sense to you, shows your child you appreciate his uniqueness and value his opinions.

A study completed in 2007 examined special interests in individuals with AS. The data showed that although the participants, who all had AS, had an overall negative self-image in other areas of their lives, they had a more positive image of themselves while they were involved in activities relating to their passion. Their knowledge and expertise about a single subject made them feel good about themselves and increased their self-confidence.

Changing Fixations

Interest in different topics can come and go. Because these fascinations are so important in the lives of Aspies, when one interest ends, it is most often replaced with another, sometimes immediately, sometimes within a few weeks. It is possible for fixations to overlap, and a child can have more than one special interest at a time. However, most times the AS child focuses on only one or two special interests at a time.

Short-term focuses may end quickly. One day your child is passionately interested in a topic, and the next day the interest is gone. Because special interests often involve collecting items relating to the interest, you end up with several different collections. Even though your child has lost interest, he may resist throwing away any of the memorabilia, feeling it still has some significance. For bright Aspies who become "a small expert on the topic" and then move on to other topics, that knowledge is not gone. After several such fixations, they become very knowledgeable on a wide variety of topics. Some, whose interests are more mainstream, can become quite well-rounded.

Simultaneous Interests

MISC.

In their book *The OASIS Guide to Asperger Syndrome,* Patty Romanowski Bashe and Barbara L. Kirby explain that some children develop two or more simultaneous interests, and the number of passions can increase as the child matures. There is frequently a "primary" interest that may come and go and bursts of intense focus on different subjects in between. These can be somewhat related, such as architecture and interior design, or completely unrelated, such as cooking and knitting.

Usually young children have one distinct special interest, often beginning with a fascination in a part of a toy, for example, playing only with the wheel of a toy truck. This can develop into a fixation with all wheels.

Lifetime Interests

Sometimes, a special interest lasts throughout a person's life. These types of preoccupations may come and go, based on whether there is new information to learn, new memorabilia to buy, or on other activities that may be taking time and focus. Your child may lose interest in something, or appear to lose interest, only to pick it back up months or years later, with passions just as high as they were before.

Lifelong interests can lead to employment opportunities. For example, a child may have an all-consuming preoccupation with computer games, learning not only the games themselves but how to design and create the game programs. This intense, sophisticated knowledge can help teens and parents narrow their search for career choices.

When Special Interests Are Inappropriate

Special interests can be about any topic. Children often become fixated on a certain cartoon, music, architecture, or famous people—the possibilities are endless. But what happens when the topic is taboo or possibly dangerous, like weapons or pornography? When this happens, parents not only worry about the immediate dangers, but the problems absorption in these types of topics causes in school. Forbidding a child with AS to be interested isn't going to work. Forbidding access may cause tantrums or sneaking to fill the need for information.

The first line of defense against such interests is to monitor what your child is exposed to in the first place. Prereading, previewing, reading reviews by other parents, and getting a sense for what the book, movie, interest, and so on involves ahead of time can yield huge unseen benefits later. If your child develops a dangerous or an inappropriate passion, see if you can find out what it is about it that appeals to your child before you rush to end it. For example, an interest in weapons could be a fascination with how a gun is made, what makes it work, or what makes one gun different than another.

After you understand the interest, you can work on guiding it toward a more appropriate focus or, if you decide it is harmless, accept it but allow only limited access. For other inappropriate passions, such as pornography, you may have to set specific rules, set up parental controls on your computer, and monitor the situation closely. It is also important to know what developmental changes are likely to be issues as your child grows. Anticipating such changes and planning for how your child is introduced to them can help shape his perspective from a potentially troublesome one to one that is more typical or appropriate.

Aspie Advice

When your child has an inappropriate special interest, rather than showing your unhappiness, remain neutral but don't participate or encourage the interest. Instead, try to steer your child to another interest. You can adopt your own special interest, reading, researching, and talking about your interest, and hope that your child will become interested as well. You can try to find an interest that is related to your child's special interest but is a more accepted topic.

Although AS is becoming more well-known, many people still don't understand it and therefore are not able to understand a child or teenager having such a strong interest in something as controversial as guns. They may assume your child is violent or be scared of your child. In these cases, if you believe the interest to be harmless, you will need to limit the interest to your own home and teach your child when it is appropriate to talk about his interest and who he is allowed to talk with about the interest.

If your child begins to focus on death or dying or is preoccupied with violence, then you may need to talk with a mental health professional. There is a high risk for depressive disorder, especially in teens with AS, and if your child's special interest begins to turn toward these types of topics, it could be a sign of depression. See Chapter 4 for more information on depression and other related conditions.

Working with Your Child's Special Interest

If you have a child with AS, there is a good chance that at some point you have been inundated with questions about his current passion. You may have planned last year's summer vacation around the special interest, and your dinner table conversation is probably dominated by facts about his fascination. When you think about what a parent can do, your first thought might be, "I want to know how to end an interest." But did you know special interests can be both motivators and learning tools? Taking the time to understand and appreciate your child's preoccupation can go a long way to finding ways to make special interests a positive experience.

Special Interests as Motivators

Tony's special interest is trains. It began when he was younger and was fascinated with Thomas the Tank Engine. Now that he is 11, he stills loves trains. Even though he still has some of his Thomas toys, they have mostly been put away, and he spends his time with a model railroad set he got last year for his birthday. He has a number of videos on trains, and every morning while eating his breakfast he watches the same one. When he gets home from school, he watches a different one.

Trains are part of Tony's everyday routine, but lately his parents have been having trouble getting him to do chores around the house. It is Tony's responsibility to take out the trash and sweep the kitchen floor. Tony's parents made up a chart listing both his chores and when they were to be completed. Each day, Tony is to mark on the chart after he finishes. At the end of the week, if he has completed his chores each day, Tony gets to take a ride on the local train. He and his parents ride the train to the next stop and then return. Most of the engineers know Tony by now and talk to him when he arrives on Saturday morning.

Tony's parents found a way to use his passion as a motivator for Tony to complete chores he didn't want to do. An added bonus was the lesson in social skills when the train engineers noticed Tony as a regular and began talking to him. Tony now had someone to share his knowledge of trains with and talked about the Saturday trips all week long.

Using special interests as a motivator works better than taking away access as a punishment. When you deny access, you can end up with a lot of frustration or anger. Sometimes parents must limit access. Using passions positively, however, can come in a variety of ways. For example, you can give your child time to interact with his interest after he has cleaned up his room or completed his homework.

The Doctor's Take

Punishing undesired behaviors is rarely more effective than rewarding desired behaviors. Punishment is very likely to result in unforeseen side effects and increases the possibility of aggression by the child. Use rewards that are frequent, consistent, and clearly defined to help change behaviors. Don't be alarmed if the undesired behaviors become worse before they become better.

Special Interests as Educational Tools

Bonny loved dogs. She spent every minute she could reading about the different breeds, and she knew where each breed originally came from. When her mom went food shopping, Bonny always went along and went directly to the pet food aisle. She would look at the different foods and read the ingredients. She knew which foods were better for young dogs and which were better for older dogs.

In school, Bonny was struggling with math. This year she was learning fractions, and she just didn't get it. Her teacher was well aware of Bonny's fascination with dogs and decided to incorporate it into the lesson. She brought in a bag of dry dog food and asked Bonny to take out enough for a dog for the entire day. She then had Bonny divide the food in half, some for the morning and some for later in the day. They did this again, pretending the dog would eat three times per day. By the end of the lesson, Bonny understood one half, one third, and one fourth, a concept she had been having a lot of difficulty with.

A Reason to Read

MISC.

Matt had no interest in reading. He didn't understand what reading could do for him. His parents and teachers tried all the normal methods of teaching Matt to read, but they all fell flat. He was evaluated for dyslexia, but testing didn't show any learning disability. Matt had a passion for all things Ford. A family friend gave him repair manuals that had the Ford logo on the front. Matt wanted to know what was in those official Ford books. Reading became necessary, and he suddenly paid attention to reading lessons. When he graduated from high school, Matt went right to work. Can you guess where?

Be creative in bringing your child's special interest into other subjects. When interacting with their passion, Aspies are more able to focus and concentrate. While math and reading most readily come to mind, there are other ways to use his favorite topic. For example, your child may watch a certain cartoon over and over. Sit with your child and use the show to talk about facial expressions or how to start a conversation.

Expanding Interests

Special interests are often narrowly focused. You can build upon that focus to incorporate additional interests and knowledge. For example, if your child is fascinated with science fiction movies, use this as a starting point to learn about the solar system or constellations.

A preoccupation with Ancient Egypt can expand into learning about other cultures, first by looking at those cultures that came into contact with Ancient Egypt and then by tracing the influences of Egypt on the development of other cultures, or by comparing and contrasting how other cultures created buildings or how they ran their governments.

Conversation Building Blocks

As any parent of a child with AS will tell you, special interests dominate conversations, so it can be a bit tricky to use them as ways to build a conversation. Start by teaching your child when and where it is appropriate to talk about his passion.

You can also teach him specific types of body language that signal a conversation partner is bored. Because of an Aspie's difficulty picking up nonverbal cues, Aspies need to be taught specific signs to look for when talking with someone. Here are some examples:

- Shuffling of feet
- Looking at a watch or looking in a different direction
- Rolling eyes
- Rubbing eyes
- Bringing up different topics

Help your child know what to do or what to say if they notice any of these actions. Some suggestions for things to say are ...

- What do you like to do?
- What did you do today?
- Enough about me, what is your favorite thing to do?

If your child is having difficulty noticing nonverbal signs and signals from others who have become bored or tired of that topic, you can develop a private signal between the two of you to use in order to let him know he needs to stop talking about the chosen topic. This has the benefit of allowing him to try to figure out when others become tired of his interest while providing a safety net for him so he doesn't go on too long and possibly alienate the listener. Private signals such as subtle gestures also have the added bonus of not calling attention to your child's difficulty with knowing when enough is enough so he can avoid embarrassment.

> **Aspie Advice**
>
> Many Aspies don't understand social cues and social language. Teach your child phrases used by children his age and to watch for gestures to help him guess what the other person is thinking. As your child matures, he will be able to grasp some of these concepts, which will go a long way to helping him feel like he fits in. Focusing on faces is a common area to start. For some, however, this makes participating in the conversation even harder. Listen when your child tells you what is hard about using nonverbal information in conversations, particularly when it comes to eye contact.

Participation in Social Functions

Depending on your child's special interest, you may be able to find a group or club in your area to help your child expand his knowledge and his social skills. If you do find a group, depending on your child's age and whether he wants to disclose his disability, you may want to talk with the group leader before your child attends. This should be a safe, secure, and fun activity, not one that is filled with teasing or bullying.

If there are no groups, you might still be able to use the special interest to help in social settings. Suppose that your child is interested in art. Is another student interested in writing? Can you or the teacher team them up to create a storybook or work on a school project together? It is often easier to find an adult who has greater knowledge and the maturity to understand your child's needs than it is to find a peer who can positively interact with him around his interest. Be careful of focusing on only adult interactions for your child. Aspies often have significantly better social skills interacting with adults, but their area of greatest need is in learning how to better interact with age-appropriate peers.

Although they're not in-person groups, you can also look for social inter-actions for your child on the internet. Interacting with others in online groups still helps to teach communication skills. When writing something in an online forum, it is usually written in a straightforward way. Humor and sarcasm may still be present, and your child may need to sometimes "read between the lines," but he will not need to try to interpret body lan-guage and can focus on the written word.

Using Special Interests to Connect

Your child may not only have problems interacting with classmates or other children. You, as his parent, may also feel a distance because of prob-lems expressing emotions or sharing happiness or sadness with others. You can use your child's special interest as a way to connect.

Take the time to play with his toys, not as you think they should be played with, but how he wants to play with them. Help him find new ways to learn about his special interest, visit the library, read books together, search for new websites, or visit a museum. Spending time with your child, on his terms, helps you appreciate and understand his passions.

Limiting Access to a Special Interest

Sometimes you must limit a child's access to a special interest to benefit either the child or the family. Without such limits, your child might ignore other responsibilities, focusing all of his time and energy on interacting with his passion. Although denying access can create tense situations, tan-trums, or meltdowns, you can limit access by using the special interest as a reward for desired behaviors.

Sometimes your child's favorite topic is dangerous. We talked earlier in the chapter about passions that are inappropriate, but sometimes the desire to find out more about a fascination may be harmful. In an earlier example, we explained Tony's special interest in trains. Once a week, if Tony com-pleted his chores, his parents took him for a ride on a train.

Imagine if Tony's insatiable quest to interact with his interest led him to take the train, without letting his parents know. He saw the train and couldn't resist the impulse to ride as he did each Saturday morning. But without his parents, Tony could get lost, not know what stop to get off, or get injured because he didn't pay attention to caution signs. Tony may not understand that his parents are at home, worried about where he is. In this case, Tony's parents would need to set strict limits on his access to train rides. It is best to talk about these issues and develop guidelines or rules with your child ahead of time. With Aspies it is easier to establish a rule or pattern than it is to correct or change an inaccurate or inappropriate one that is already established.

> **The Doctor's Take**
>
> When limiting access to a special interest, keep in mind how important the passion is and think about how it helps in your child's development and helps him feel secure. Instead of taking away or limiting an interest, try to make a trade. Offer extra time interacting with the favorite topic if he joins a club at school or agrees to participate in some social function.

You also might have practical reasons for setting limits. If a special interest is a movie, your child might collect action figures, cards, and other memorabilia. If an item is broken or lost, you may need to replace the item. Sometimes, such as Tony's train rides each Saturday, you spend money to help your child pursue and learn about his passion. Financial restraints may require parents to place limits on how much money is spent on trinkets.

When other children are in the family, time spent on the special interest may need to be limited in order to make sure each child feels valued and appreciated. Family dinner conversations cannot be dominated by one child and one topic. As parents, you need to make time to talk with each child. At these times, you need to set specific rules about when or for how long the family discussions will be about a single topic. Your Aspie needs to learn respect for all members of the family. This is a perfect opportunity to teach turn-taking, sharing, and general rules for balancing the needs of one person with those of the rest of the family.

It is sometimes hard for an Aspie to give up on a passion, even if it is childish. For example, a child may have developed a fascination with Thomas the Tank Engine as a young child but can't seem to let it go. Now that he is in school, some of the other children are starting to tease him because he still watches the show each day. Your child may naturally try to hide his preoccupation from his classmates, showing the class more grown-up trains, but you can let your child continue to pursue it at home. You can also encourage more mature ways to continue, such as looking for collectible items on online auctions. This allows your child to continue his special interest without the teasing.

Essential Takeaways

- Special interests are very common and can be a potential source of stress relief for your child.

- Monitoring passions, anticipating possible problems, and helping your child incorporate his interests productively into his life can result in his harnessing his fascination to learn a great deal.

- Some Aspies continue a single interest throughout their lives and use this topic in their career choice.

- Because passions can be about any topic, they are sometimes inappropriate, such as an interest in guns or pornography. Parents can help by limiting access or help shape the fascination into a more typical or appropriate interest.

chapter 9

Special Interests Through the Years

Early interests in objects rather than topics

Young children's attachment to items in a collection

Video games as a passion in early adolescence

Special interests as part of your teen's identity

Special interests are one of the hallmark signs of Asperger's syndrome (AS). These interests are similar to interests and hobbies in those without AS, but differ in intensity. Interests may begin in early childhood and last throughout your child's lifetime. Although not all children with AS have a passionate interest, the majority develop such interests.

The Early Years

As early as 2 or 3 years old, your child may have shown intense interest in different parts of toys rather than playing with the toys as intended. For example, Jack's aunt and uncle brought a toy dump truck for Christmas. Jack sat down with the truck and examined it. His aunt sat down and rolled the truck, making "vroom" noises, but Jack was more interested in making the back of the truck go up and down. He spent the next hour turning the switch to raise the truck bed and then bringing it back down. Often, a young Aspie is fascinated by parts of objects, spinning wheels, or turning something off and on.

From Early Interests to Career

Billy started off interested in Thomas the Tank Engine, and he learned everything there was to know about the topic; later he became passionate about real trains and again learned everything he could. As Billy got older his passion included freight, which led him to investigate logistics and how things are efficiently moved from one location to another. Ultimately Billy got a degree in business logistics and now works at improving the flow of freight at his company.

Your child might be more interested in the patterns, letters, or numbers on the blocks than on using the blocks to build. He might find that intricate pattern on the cover of the book much more fascinating than the book itself. After he notices an object, he may not be able to pay attention to anything else. At the early ages, he is interested more in objects than in topics.

By the time your child becomes a toddler, he may have developed an intense interest in a single topic. Many young boys with AS take an interest in Thomas the Tank Engine, but interests are varied, and it could be as different as a fascination with pots and pans. Even at the age of 4, your child wants to learn as much as possible about his interest. He will ask questions incessantly, look at books, and watch videos. He has a high motivation to learn. For example, your child may strive to learn to read so he can learn about his passion. A child fascinated with numbers may be able to count well beyond what other children his age are counting. He may use vocabulary specific to his interest and show a high level of expertise, especially for such a young child.

Early Elementary Age

If your child has not yet started to move from an interest in objects to an interest in topics, at this age he will become more and more interested in a specific topic. For boys with AS, topics of interest usually revolve around science and transportation, such as trains, trucks, dinosaurs, electronics, or space. Your child may be interested in sports, but not necessarily to play; instead he is fascinated with statistics, facts, and players. He may know every team in a league and be able to name every player on each team. Because of his insatiable curiosity about the topic, he can develop an encyclopedic knowledge.

> **The Doctor's Take**
>
> Although most Aspies develop narrowly focused interests, not all do. Some children with AS do not develop a focal interest at all, and others seem to go through a series of intense interests. One of the hardest things with diagnosing AS is that each child has a different combination of issues relating to restricted and stereotyped patterns or interests. But remember, the lack of mastery or passion of a single topic does not rule out AS.

Some other common topics of interest include:

- *Types of workers.* Your child may be fascinated with policemen, firemen, or plumbers. He may dress up in costume, wearing it to the store, restaurants, or to school.

- *Animals.* He may be interested in a specific animal, such as a dog, horse, or a butterfly. Your child may pretend to be the animal.

- *Dinosaurs.* Although no living dinosaurs are available to study, the accumulation of facts and figures is a perfect way to master this area. This is one of the more common passionate interests for AS children.

Although your child may pretend to be the object of their interest, they don't usually make up scenarios and stories, but rather act out realistic scenes or mimic actions seen on television or depicted in a book.

During this stage, your child may begin collecting items. Just like interests, these collections are as varied as children with AS. Collections can range from milk bottle caps, paper clips, pencils, golf balls, or stones. Collections, as with interests, are solitary activities; your child doesn't need and often doesn't want other people involved, except as a source of information. Your child will know every piece in his collection, he will see the different colors, the imperfections, and all other visual characteristics. He will know and be upset if a piece is missing and will spend time searching for new items to add to the collection. He may seem as if he has an attachment or affection for the items in his collection. For some this attachment is more readily expressed than his feeling of attachment for his own family.

Most of your child's conversations will begin with his favorite topic. He will hold one-sided conversations, not aware that others don't have the same level of interest or don't want to hear about the topic. These interests can intrude into the classroom, resulting in your child disrupting the class, interrupting the teacher, talking incessantly about his interest, or not paying attention to lessons because he is focusing on his passion.

Preteen Years

During early adolescence, special interests continue to dominate your child's life and his conversations. Your child is trying to understand the changing social relationships as peers focus more on personalities than activities. He may feel lost and isolated and become even more engulfed in his passion. Many children become more and more preoccupied with video or computer games during this stage. These games give them an opportunity to interact with other people, without the challenge of face-to-face interactions.

The Doctor's Take	Creating different collections can continue into preteen, teen, and adult years. Many times, even when your child is no longer interested in adding to a collection, he won't want to throw anything out. This can result in having numerous collections, of varying sizes and items, all around your child's room or throughout the house.

Communication in online chat rooms relies on short, typed questions and responses. Body language is not required, and your child may feel comfortable with this type of social interaction. He doesn't need to guess about facial expressions or look for other nonverbal cues; he simply needs to read the text and respond. When a question is asked, he can take his time responding, thinking about what he wants to say. He can relax and have fun without the pressure of face-to-face interactions.

You must explain possible dangers in participating in online sites and put rules in place in order to protect your child. If your child learns better through video modeling, which is common for Aspies, a number of videos have been produced that do an excellent job of appropriately spelling out the dangers of online social interactions and lay out good ground rules for participating. Two excellent online resources are:

- "Internet Safety—A Parent's Guide to the Internet," a PowerPoint presentation by the New York Department of Criminal Justice, can be found at http://criminaljustice.state.ny.us/missing/i_safety/videos_presentations.htm.

- John Walsh's Safe Side series is available at www.thesafeside.com.

Video games offer a way to escape from real life. Many games mimic social interactions but without the pressure of doing everything right. Your child can make mistakes and learn, without pressure. The games are predictable. If he follows the rules (which he does), then certain outcomes occur. These games also give your child the repetition and consistency he needs in his life to feel secure.

Whether your child's passion revolves around video games or washing machines, in the preteen and teen years, the pressure of the outside world can drive your child to spend more and more time with the interest. He may withdraw from real-life situations because they are too difficult and too stressful. You are left trying to create a balance. Even though special interests help your child cope, there is the chance of "too much of a good thing." One way to balance his time is to use his passion as a reward. For example, you may say, "After your homework is completed, you can play your video games for one hour." Or you may want to encourage outside activities, giving your child extra time to interact with his interest if he agrees to join a club at school.

The Teen Years

During the teen years children both with and without AS are "finding their identities." They are trying to figure out who they are and how they fit into the world. Your child probably associates his interests with his identity. For example, when asked to describe themselves, teens without AS may use words like "friendly," "nice," or "smart." If your child has developed an extraordinary amount of information on baseball statistics, he may describe himself as "an expert on baseball" rather than naming various personality traits. His interests, in his mind, help make up who he is.

Nerds and Geeks

Misc.

Some teens with AS seem to have a natural ability to understand computer language and have advanced programming skills. Many teens with AS may be seen as nerds or geeks. Because they can solve peers' computer problems or access cheat codes in video games, they may earn the respect of their classmates. There is even an autobiography written by a tween with AS titled *Freaks, Geeks, and Asperger's Syndrome!*

Frequently, your child's favorite topics are the same interests he had as a young child. In a previous section we discussed Thomas the Tank Engine being a common passion for young boys. It would not be unusual for a teen to still be fascinated with this interest. If your teen has carried a special interest throughout his young life, you need to be aware of how this may be perceived by his classmates. Most will not understand and, if they knew, may ridicule your child for being interested in "baby" shows.

Explain to your teen that you do not have a problem with his favorite topic, and as long as he is in the house, he can watch the videos or use the toys. Explain how it may look to others and talk about when he should and should not talk about it. List places it is okay to discuss the interest so that others will not overhear and tease him. List people who he can trust to talk to and who might share his passion.

If your teen has an interest that is young for his age, think about other ways he can pursue the interest without appearing too immature. Using the example of Thomas the Tank Engine, go online with your teen and look for collectibles. He may enjoy finding out about the different collectible items, how much they are worth, and what they are projected to be worth in the future. This helps your teen use his passion and expand his interests, learning about the world of "collectibles."

Some teens with AS find their interests move from objects to people. They can become fascinated with a pop star, a movie star, or someone in your neighborhood. As with all special interests, your teen wants to know as much as possible about his interest. He will read online articles, search for trivia and facts, want to watch the movies, or go to the concerts. This can be concerning if the person your teen is fascinated with is someone in your neighborhood, someone their own age, or a teacher. He will still strive to find out everything he can about the person, but his actions can be misinterpreted, and he could be viewed as a stalker. Let your teen know what is appropriate and what is not appropriate.

Beyond the Teen Years

As we have previously discussed, special interests are often a foundation for career choices; for example, a fascination with computers can lead to employment in software development or computer repair. For many, this single-mindedness allows Aspies to develop a high level of knowledge about a particular topic, commonly science or math, and excel in their jobs. Other adults with AS may find teaching a great job; not only can they use the knowledge they have about a topic, they can share it with others.

Essential Takeaways

- Special interests may be noticed as early as 2 or 3 years old but often begin as a preoccupation with an object, or a part of an object, rather than a topic.
- Collections are as varied as passions and can be milk bottle caps, paper clips, or stones. Your child will know every piece in the collection and know when a piece is missing.
- Many preteens and teens are interested in electronics, video games, or computer games as their passion.
- Teens can closely align their identity with their special interest.

Social Skills

The most difficult area for children with Asperger's syndrome (AS) is in social skills. In Part 4, we help you understand how the symptoms of AS can interfere with playing with other children, making friends, keeping friends, and learning about relationships.

We explain social skills challenges throughout an Aspie's life, beginning with parallel and copycat playing in the early years and the need to define personal spaces and the downside of total honesty in elementary school. We talk about the more mature friendships and relationships of the teen years.

Aspies are often targets of bullies, and we discuss how parents can recognize the signs that your child might be the victim of a bully. We offer tips on working with the school to create an antibullying program and educate teachers to spot and stop bullying in the classroom and on the recess yard.

Social skills difficulties continue for young adults with AS, and we provide information for managing AS in the workplace, including navigating different relationships such as co-workers and supervisors. As a young adult, your child will sometimes need to disclose his diagnosis, and we talk about ways to prepare him for talking about AS. Finally, we discuss different types of living arrangements for young adults and explain the pros and cons of each.

chapter 10

Social Competence

Three important components of social skills

Learning to join in conversations

Distinguishing friends from acquaintances

Improving your child's social skills

Social skills are a combination of skills that help people communicate, relate, and form emotional connections with one another. They can differ depending on your family dynamics, your cultural and religious beliefs, and your expectations of social relationships. In this chapter, we'll discuss different skills involved in social competence and give tips on how you can help your child.

What Are Social Skills?

Getting along with others, asking for help, making and keeping friends, and developing romantic relations all require social skills. Children with Asperger's syndrome (AS) have a difficult time mastering these skills and lack social "common sense," which makes it hard for them to relate to other children and make friends. Some of the common components of social skills include:

Verbal communication. Knowing what to say and when to say it, speaking with inflection and being able to talk so others can understand what you mean.

Nonverbal communication. Understanding facial expressions and body language and the emotion behind words or understanding what has been implied or inferred.

Listening skills. Being able to actively listen while other people speak and process this information quickly enough to respond appropriately.

Children with AS tend think in literal, concrete terms. Social skills are abstract concepts, which makes them hard for your child to understand. For example, telling your child to "be nice" or "show kindness" likely has absolutely no meaning to them. Instead, you will need to give specific instructions on what behavior constitutes "nice" or "kind."

Understanding Emotion

There is a belief that Aspies lack *empathy*. Although your child may sometimes seem unaware of others' feelings, it is most likely because he doesn't understand the emotion behind the words. He probably has difficulty reading expressions on the other person's face, and because he thinks in such a literal way, is often challenged by humor, sarcasm, or implied meaning.

> **Empathy** is the ability to implicitly identify and understand another person's feelings and motives and to respond accordingly.
>
> Definition

Reading Faces

From the time they are young, children seem to instinctively sense a parent's mood and react accordingly. As children grow and mature, they are able to distinguish moods based on the look on their parent's face. Your child either struggles with this or just can't do this. He will use spoken words to derive what other people feel, but words alone don't always tell the whole story. You will need to work with your child to help him read emotion on people's faces.

One way to help your child is to create an "emotions book." Focus on one emotion at a time, such as "happy." Use a binder or scrapbook and look through books (that you don't mind cutting up) or magazines and cut out pictures of people looking happy. During the time you are working on this emotion, sing songs, read stories, watch videos, and point out people in public to show your child a range of expressions that show someone is happy. You want to point out different levels of being happy, from mildly happy to ecstatic, as your child may not understand the differences, assuming everyone who is happy feels the same level of emotion.

Your child may also have a problem showing emotion on his face. Some Aspies, when asked to make a "happy" face, will use their fingers to move their lips into a smile. Some can do one emotion but not others, and for boys, the most common one that is mastered is anger. Use a mirror to help him practice making faces to show emotion. In the beginning, you may need to exaggerate showing emotion on your face to help him understand what you are feeling. Here are some additional ideas and games to play with your child:

- Create a "Mr. Potato Head" game, making up different eyes and mouths that show happiness, anger, frustration, and sadness. Attach fasteners to a cardboard face where the eyes and mouth belong and fasteners to the back of each piece. When you state an emotion, your child needs to find the right eyes and mouth to convey that feeling.

- Write down different emotions on index cards. Pin one card on someone's back so they can't see which emotion is written down and get other members of the family to act out that emotion. The person with the index card tries to guess the emotion. Have everyone take turns guessing the emotion. Your Aspie learns how to both recognize and display emotions.

- Have your child keep a diary. Sometimes it is easier for your child to write down emotions than to verbally explain them. Writing down how they feel helps them better identify their own emotions in other situations.

Still Waters Run Deep

Misc.

Joe was referred to as "inscrutable" because his face generally had a neutral expression. However, Joe could feel emotion, and many often overlooked this fact because of his calm external demeanor. One day, a new student was teasing Joe and got a surprise when Joe's expression showed full rage. His face was animated, his skin was red, and he raised his voice. The new student was shocked, but the kids who had known Joe for years were not. His teacher told the new boy that "still waters run deep."

When your child has made significant progress in recognizing facial expressions and being able to show that emotion on his face, move to another emotion. If you have created a scrapbook or binder for each emotion, as you complete one emotion, take one or two pages and place in a new binder so your child has an expanded scrapbook for each emotion and a "reference" book to flip through to see different emotions.

Talk to your child about appropriate reactions to each emotion. When he is recognizing sadness on someone's face, it is okay to say, "I am sorry that you are feeling sad." Understanding that other people feel different emotions is the first step toward developing empathy.

Recognizing Body Language and Tone of Voice

Just as your child has trouble recognizing and using facial expressions, she doesn't accurately read body language. How we hold our bodies and use our hands when interacting with another person can give many clues to how we are feeling. How something is said and the tone used also tells a lot about what the speaker means. Without this understanding, words can take on a whole different meaning for a child with AS.

Mary was unaware of her body language and had struggled with the concept. Things seemed to be getting more and more complicated each year. When she was in elementary school, no one seemed to misunderstand her—at least that is what she thought. Now in middle school, it was all so complicated. Why did the boys think she was giving them permission to touch her? Her therapist and mom kept telling her that she was standing too close and leaning into the boys too much. So?! She'd done that all her life, why was it an issue now? Wasn't it the boys who had changed? Mary was certain that she hadn't!

Your child needs to understand that just as she needs to learn body language to help understand what the other person is trying to convey, she also needs to know how to use body language to help others understand the meaning behind her words. It's also important as parents to remember that as children grow and mature, body language changes; for example, a young child may jump up and down to show excitement, while an older child may show their excitement through facial expression. As a parent, you need to continually teach body language that is common in their current age group.

The Doctor's Take	When someone you are speaking to does not make eye contact, you think he is not interested, not paying attention, or not telling the truth. When explaining how to make eye contact to your child, be specific; he may not understand "make eye contact," as this is an abstract thought. Instead, make a red arrow and point to your eye so he learns where to look. Use the words "point your eyes" instead of "make eye contact."

There are many ways to interpret body language, and none of us gets it right all of the time. However, some fairly universal gestures hold specific meanings that you can explain to your child:

- *Arms crossed, pointing whole body away from the speaker.* This usually signals that someone is closed to your ideas or is not interested in what you have to say.

- *Leaning forward, tilting head, arms open, face pointed directly at the speaker.* This shows the listener is interested in what you have to say.

- *Tapping toes, swinging feet, drumming fingers.* Usually this signals boredom on the part of the listener.

- *Clenched fists, flushed face, holding body rigid.* Clearly signals anger or frustration.

- *Waving hands, using hands when talking.* Signals excitement—can be happy excitement, frustration, or possibly anger.

As you and your child watch how others react, either in person or on television, add body language cues to your list. Your child can refer to the list when he is confused about how someone is feeling. Remember to let him know that body language can mean different things in different cultures as well.

> **Nonverbal Communication**
>
> misc.
>
> Only 7 percent of communication is based on words; tone of voice accounts for 38 percent and body language for another 55 percent. All three must be present for effective communication to take place, according to Albert Mehrabian, Professor Emeritus of Psychology at UCLA.

Tone of voice and inflections while speaking also tell a great deal about the meaning behind the words. A raised voice can indicate excitement or anger. A soft voice can indicate shyness, insecurity, or that someone is not sure about what he is saying.

Peter was 5 years old and had been sitting at the table drawing for several hours. His lunch was sitting next to him, untouched. When his mother came into the room, she exclaimed, "Peter, you haven't touched your lunch. You were supposed to eat. I made your favorite sandwich over an hour ago!" Because Peter's mother had raised her voice, most children would understand that she was upset, but Peter did not. He said, "I wasn't hungry yet, but why are you talking in your outside voice when we are inside?" Peter heard only the words and responded to them.

The most effective way to teach social skills is through modeling behavior, role-playing, and giving your child plenty of opportunities to practice. Peter's mother used the situation to talk to Peter about how someone's voice changes based on their emotion. She modeled saying the same sentence in several different ways. One time she sounded worried that something was wrong because Peter had not eaten. Once she showed surprise, and another time she said the same words but sounded angry. She wanted Peter to hear how emotion can change the meaning of the words.

Inferring Meaning

Sarcasm, humor, figures of speech, and idioms are all problem areas that can interfere with your child's ability to make friends. In Chapter 6, we talked about how your child interprets language literally, having a hard time when figures of speech are thrown into conversations. Your child's confusion or inappropriate responses make him seem "odd" or different, and his classmates may shy away from him.

Ronny was in middle school, and one of his classmates, George, was talking to him about a video game. Ronny had already completed the level that George was working on. George wanted some hints on how to get past a certain point, and he knew that Ronny was the person to ask. Their classmates called Ronny "the video game genius" and often came to him for help. George listened carefully to what Ronny said, and as he was leaving said, "Thanks, Ronny, catch you later." Ronny was confused; what did George mean? Was George going to chase him home? What was going to happen when George caught him? From then on, Ronny avoided George, afraid that George was going to do something bad to him.

> **The Doctor's Take**
>
> Classmates and other children may say mean things to your child. Be sure to teach reactions that are less likely to get your child in trouble or increase the chances that the other children will keep saying those things to him—for example, walking away, laughing, or talking to an adult. Giving your child a "menu" of different reactions to choose from may stop him from reacting aggressively and ending up in trouble.

Humor and teasing are another way literal thinking interferes with relationships. Teasing each other is one way children connect with one another, a way to express that you like the other person and you accept them, faults and all. Suppose that George had said to Ronny, "Wow, you are so great at video games, don't you wish you were that good at math?" and then laughed. Ronny, not understanding, might reply with, "But I am good at math," or "Yes, I do wish that." Ronny's odd response could have George shaking his head. Sometimes teasing isn't so neutral, and your child might take teasing statements the wrong way, becoming angry or aggressive. His inability to understand the teasing sets him apart from the other kids and makes him feel disconnected from his classmates.

Holding Conversations

Your child may talk nonstop about his interest or shy away from joining in conversations. Both can be immense barriers to making friends. Teaching your child the art of conversation is a tough job. Not only does he need to know how to start and end a conversation but how to respond in the middle to keep it going. Help your child by giving him options to choose from.

Conversation Starters

- Hello or hi.

- How are you doing?

- What's up?

- What are you doing after school today?

- What did you do last night/over the weekend/over the summer?

Aspie Advice

In addition to giving your child a list of ideas for conversation feedback, teach him that body language, such as nodding his head, keeping his face pointed toward the person speaking, and being still while the person is talking, helps to convey that he is interested in the conversation.

Conversation Feedback

- That's interesting/neat/cool.

- I don't know what you mean; could you explain that?

- That's great.

- What did you do then?

- I am sorry to hear that.

Conversation Ends

- I'll catch you later.

- See you later/tomorrow/next week/Monday.

- Bye.

- I have to go now.

If your child tends to butt into the conversation, teach him phrases such as:

- May I add to what you are saying?
- Is it okay if I say something?
- Excuse me, could I add something?

Some of these phrases won't be appropriate for your child's age or maturity level. Watch videos, observe other children together, and read books to add age-appropriate phrases for him. After you do that, role-play different conversations to show him how to use the phrases during a conversation.

Understanding Different Relationships

Your child is going to meet many different people, in school, through community programs, or in your neighborhood. It may be hard for your son to understand that relationships are different depending on the person. Once he learns the rules for friendship, he may assume those rules apply to every person he meets. Poor social skills include being too familiar with those you don't know yet. For example, your child can sit close to you on a couch, but it may be awkward when he stands way too close to a stranger or acquaintance, ignoring *personal space*. You also must protect your child from danger by making sure he knows the difference between a friend and a stranger and what types of conversations and behaviors are appropriate with each group.

Definition

Personal space is the area immediately surrounding someone, usually around 3 feet, in which that person feels threatened or uncomfortable when someone enters into this space.

In Chapter 3, we offered a tip of creating a relationship circle. In the innermost circle, your family members are listed along with appropriate behavior and conversation topics. The next circle represents relatives, the third circle represents friends, the fourth represents acquaintances, and the last represents strangers. For each circle, list people you know and behaviors, as you did with family members. When your child meets someone new, help him to place that person in the right category. Explain to him that sometimes people move from one category to another; for example, an acquaintance can become a friend.

Tips to Help Build Social Competence

Teaching social skills to Aspies is an ongoing process. Make sure you explain concepts in concrete terms. The phrase "personal space" is an abstract and relative term; use "one arm's length" instead to give your child a specific way to measure space when talking to someone. Arm your child with if-then rules to help with social manners. For example, if someone says "thank you," then he should say "you are welcome."

Besides specific social actions, you need to continually discuss friendship and social interaction. Reading books about these topics and talking about the story with your child provides examples of what a friend is and how friends treat one another. You can also model social behavior and talk aloud about what you are doing, such as talking with the cashier at the store or meeting a friend on the street. Explain what you did and why. Finally, be sure to create opportunities for your child to practice social skills at home. Invite one child over after school where you can monitor how your child interacts.

Essential Takeaways

- Children with AS do not necessarily lack empathy; they may not be able to discern the other person's feelings and therefore can't react to them.

- Teaching common body language, such as what it means if someone crosses her arms or taps her toes while conversing, will help your child learn how to pay attention to both the words being spoken and how they are being spoken.

- Figures of speech and idioms, such as "I'll catch you later" are confusing to children with AS. Make sure to keep a list of current and trendy phrases for your child to learn.

- Being able to communicate well includes understanding different types of relationships and what types of topics to talk about with each group.

chapter 11

Asperger's Syndrome in Young Children

Differences in Aspies' play activities

Helping your child develop flexibility in play

What is reciprocal play?

Including other children in play

Play is an important part of your child's development. The American Academy of Pediatrics states that play provides benefits for "cognitive, social, emotional, physical, and moral development." Your child's play may not look or feel like the play of other children. Your child may line up toys or be preoccupied with parts of toys rather than the whole toy. He may use toys in ways different than what they were created for. He may also lack the ability to engage in imaginative play. Early Intervention (EI) programs use a variety of therapists to help children with Asperger's syndrome (AS) develop play skills, but as a parent, you can work with your child more often during playtime.

Parallel Play vs. Cooperative Play

In typical child development, at around 2 years old, your child plays by himself, with little awareness of others as "people." Children at this age follow simple directions and play based on an adult's guidance; for example, he will roll a car if you roll a car and then hand it to him and ask him to do the same. By the time he turns 3, solitary play turns into parallel play. Your child enjoys being around other children, and if playing cars will sit on the floor next to another child. Their play, however, will usually be separate, each child playing in their own way.

Around the age of 4, a child begins *cooperative play* and may seek out other children to play with. He can participate in group games, such as duck-duck-goose. Playing with other children includes talking and the simple sharing of ideas. For example, a child might say, "Let's do it this way." Cooperative play continues to develop, and by the age of 5, he has favorite playmates and can play games that require taking turns. Your child may stay in the solitary play stage well past the age when other children have moved on to cooperative play.

Definition

Cooperative play refers to play in which children plan and assign roles to one another, for example, when children play house and divide up chores. This type of play usually has a goal or specific end, is more organized than play seen in younger years, and includes learning how to take turns. This type of play continues throughout the elementary school years.

Chandra was thrilled to find a playgroup at her local church. She was a stay-at-home mom and thought her son Kevin, age 4, needed other children to play with. On the first day, Kevin surveyed the room and found a toy train, an engine and five cars. He picked it up, sat down in the corner, put the cars all in line, rolled it around, took it apart, and put the cars back together again. He did the same thing over and over while the other children sat close together in a group, playing on the floor.

Chandra noticed Kevin by himself, and it reinforced her belief that he spent too much time alone with her. She thought he just needed time to get used to having other children around. But six months later, Kevin was still content to sit by himself with the toy train. The only time he got upset was when they arrived late and someone else was playing with the train. He would throw a tantrum, and as much as Chandra would try to give him a different toy and calm him down, it never worked. On those days, Chandra made up an excuse to leave early and imagined the other mothers were just as happy that she had left.

Copycat vs. Imaginative Play

Mike, at age 6, was interested in Thomas the Tank Engine. His shelves had lines of train engines and cars. He had tracks lined up on one shelf, and there were several playsets sitting on the floor. He spent hours playing with the trains, usually acting out an entire episode of the show, word for word. He never deviated from the script.

> **Aspie Advice**
>
> Have a variety of toys available for your child to choose from that help build imaginative skills as well as improve other skills. Puzzles, bean bags, and Play-Dough all help develop fine motor skills. Play keyboards and dot-to-dot drawing help visual focus. Blocks and Legos help develop spatial relationship skills. Consider having several different sets of toys you can rotate to help reduce resistance to change and increase flexibility.

Some children with AS do use creative or imaginative play, but much like Mike, their play is based on a script—one they read, saw on television, or made up. They frequently repeat the same script day after day. Here are some steps to help your child learn new ways to play:

1. Choose a toy your child regularly plays with.

2. Find out how other children would use this toy. If you have other children, nieces or nephews, or have access to a children's play-group, bring the toy along (without your child) and observe how other children play with the toy.

3. Have your child play with the toy and see how his play is different than the other children.

4. Sit with your child and show him another way to play with the toy, introducing one new way at a time.

5. Give the toy back to your child and ask him to use it the way you did.

6. Continue the same way until your child is comfortable using the toy in the acceptable way.

Here's an example of this process:

Aaron had a collection of matchbox cars. His usual play consisted of choosing 10 cars and lining them up in a particular order, and then selecting 10 more and lining them up. Betsy, his mother, already knew that other children played with the cars by rolling them along on the floor, crashing them into one another, and building roads and ramps for the cars. They also pushed two cars on the road, racing them to see which one was faster. She sat on the floor with the cars and chose one that Aaron had not yet selected. She pushed the car, making a "vroom" noise as she pushed. She handed Aaron the car and asked him to push the car. At first he took the car and lined it up next to the others, but Betsy told him she wanted to make that car move. Finally, Aaron copied his mother's behavior and pushed the car while making noise.

The next day, Betsy propped up a book to create a ramp and rolled a car down the ramp. She handed Aaron the car and, with less prodding than the previous day, he rolled the car down the ramp. Betsy continued working on these two ways to use the cars until Aaron felt comfortable and included them in his play.

Copycat play, such as acting out a script from a television show or, as Aaron did, copying his mother's behavior, helps to teach your child to have greater flexibility in his thinking and that it is okay to use an object in more than one way. Betsy continued working with Aaron so that when he went to school, his play more closely resembled the play of other children.

Reciprocal Play

Reciprocal play is when two or more children play together and both receive some benefit from the play. Reciprocal play doesn't normally begin until around 4 years old, but you have been engaging in reciprocal behavior with your child since he was an infant. Sharing a smile or imitating facial expressions are the beginnings of reciprocal actions. Although your child may not appear to react to you in the same way as children without AS, there is much research to show that Aspies do respond to reciprocal actions.

Many people describe reciprocal play as give-and-take, sharing, or taking turns, but it is more than that. Reciprocity involves two people relating on the same level, as equals. When one person is guiding and one person following, it is not reciprocal play. You can help your child by applying reciprocity in your daily interactions. Many play strategies, including the steps outlined in the previous section, help to teach your child to play with a toy in a different way than he usually does by having him copy your behavior. To help him learn reciprocal play, you want to start by mimicking his behavior.

> **The Doctor's Take**
>
> Help your child to understand what it means to be "bossy." This can help them in two very important and distinct ways: first, it can help them avoid being "bossy" with their friends and playmates, and second, it can help them accurately identify those children who are being "bossy" toward them.

A specific type of play therapy, Floortime, uses reciprocal play as a way to aid in development. You can use the principles of this type of therapy in your home. Set aside some time each day to play without you giving guided instructions. Instead, follow your child's lead. Play with the toy he wants to play with, the way he wants to play. The goal in this type of play is to take his normally solitary play and make it a joint effort, one in which you interact and connect with one another. You will use his form of play and interject ways that foster interaction.

Sam was sitting on the floor with his cars. His mother sat down next to him and asked if she could play, too. She asked for a car, and Sam gave her a green one. Sam was rolling his car on the floor, and his mother rolled her car on the floor for a few minutes. Sam continued rolling his car but would occasionally look over to see what his mother was doing. She put down the green car and asked if she could have a red one instead, Sam picked up a red car and gave it to her. His mother continued to play with the car, but would add in ways to foster interaction, such as blocking Sam's car with hers or asking him about what he was doing. As Sam's mother continued playing with Sam, on his terms, each day, he started interacting more and more often and his solitary play was turning into reciprocal play.

Continue to add words to your play, commenting on what is going on rather than giving your child directions. For example, you might say, "Look at how this car goes so much faster than this one." As your child builds his ability to engage in reciprocal play, you can include another child, asking a sibling or neighbor to join you. Sit with both children, including both in your conversation, such as asking both "I really like the red car better, what color car do you like best?" Point out different emotions; for example, "Look, John is really happy playing with you, Sam. Do you see how he is smiling?"

Aspie Advice	Sitting on the floor for extended periods of time can be hard for children with sensory sensitivities. Layer several blankets on the floor to make it softer or have a special "floor pillow" to make sitting on the floor more comfortable.

Your child may be confused by other children's play behavior. John may take several cars and race them around. Use this as an opportunity to explain different ways to play with cars without giving direct instruction. Instead, use simple language to explain, "Look what John is doing. He is racing the two cars. Which one do you think is faster?" This helps to draw your child into John's play.

As with all methods of teaching Aspies, be patient. In the beginning, you may find yourself giving your child direction instead of following his lead because you are used to "teaching through instruction." Remind yourself that during your playtime, you are focusing on your child's interests and learning more about what he thinks and wants. Even if you don't initially see any progress, continue using reciprocal play techniques every day. A study completed by Geraldine Dawson and Larry Galpert in 1990 showed that using these techniques dramatically increases eye contact and creative behavior.

Essential Takeaways

- Your child may continue with solitary play long after other children have moved on to cooperative play.

- You can help your child be more flexible by showing him how to use toys in different ways.

- Reciprocal play is when two or more children play together and both receive enjoyment from the activity.

- Floortime is one type of play therapy that helps teach Aspies how to play with other children.

chapter 12

Improving Social Skills in Elementary Age Children

Why Aspies are bossy or controlling

Learning to respect personal space

Being honest to a fault

Tips to help children ask to play

To the observer, a child with Asperger's syndrome (AS) appears selfish; however, self-centered would be a more appropriate term. Many are not motivated or interested in joining social situations or making friends. Those who are interested may not know how to talk to other children or join in their play. In this chapter, we go over some of the ways AS interferes with a child's ability to make and keep friends and give ideas on how you can help.

Learning to Interact and Communicate with Others

Katherine invited a classmate, Jenny, to play dolls at her house on Sunday. In the morning, Katherine was excited and got all of her dolls, houses, and accessories out and laid them on the floor. She took time to categorize the dolls—the ones with brown hair were in one area, the ones with blond in another. The accessories were laid out neatly—hats all together, dresses laid out according to color, shoes and other accessories placed in another area, also lined up according to color. Katherine had several videos about the dolls, but her favorite was one about two girls visiting a castle and rescuing a friend. Katherine often had her dolls act out the entire episode, word for word, and was planning that she and Jenny do it together.

> **Aspie Advice**
>
> If your child has a special or favorite toy he doesn't want to share, put that toy away before another child comes over to play. You will avoid having your child get upset because his friend is using the "wrong" toy. Remember, adults do the same thing when company comes over—this is not uniquely an AS strategy, even if it may be more important for a child with AS.

Jenny arrived, and Katherine showed her all of the dolls and accessories. Jenny immediately picked up a doll and wanted to dress her in a fancy outfit. Katherine grabbed the clothes from Jenny and gave her the "right" clothes to put on the doll. Jenny didn't understand why they needed to act out the video. She wanted to make up what the dolls were going to do. Katherine kept telling Jenny what to do and what the dolls should be doing. Jenny kept picking up dolls, changing outfits, and making up a new storyline. Katherine got angry, and the play date ended when she refused to play with Jenny.

Your child, like Katherine, may be bossy when playing with other children. She wants to play with other children, as long as they play according to her rules. When the other child wants to follow her own play rules, your child gets angry or simply stops playing. Although this seems to others as if she is controlling, her play rules are important. These rules provide a sense of security for her. When she follows her rules, she knows exactly what will happen; she knows how to react; she feels safe. There are no surprises and no situations that cause her to feel inadequate or in which she won't know what to say. This is why it is very important to ask your child what her expectations are prior to a new or unusual event. Listening to what she is expecting gives you the information you need to plan and help her effectively navigate the new situations with less chance of having serious problems.

Solitary Time vs. Developing Friendships

misc.

During the elementary school ages, your child may not be motivated to play with others, preferring to be by himself. Although it is beneficial to make sure your child is allowed solitary playtime, it is also important to encourage developing friendships. Later, during the teen years and beyond, your child may want to create social connections, and the skills you teach during the early years provides him with the ability to develop and maintain friendships.

In Chapter 11, we covered helping your child find new ways to play with toys and how to introduce him to reciprocal play, where all participants contribute to and enjoy the activity. You can continue to work with your child, introducing small changes in play routines and explaining that play isn't "wrong" if it is done in a different way. Before inviting another child over, go over the rules, and set some limits. For example, ask the other child if he wants to do it this way and set a time limit before he has to try it the other child's way. In the earlier years, you will need to stay with your child when a friend is over to help foster interaction and sharing. The more successful the initial outing, the better the chance your child's new friend will want to return. As your child gets older, staying with them for an outing can pose a problem for them socially. Begin monitoring play dates early while having Mommy or Daddy around to cue them isn't seen as weird or smothering.

Specific Childhood Behaviors

In Chapter 10, we discussed some of the main obstacles to social interactions for children with AS. The following sections address some of the issues that are more common to elementary age children. As children grow up, the social expectations of adults and their peers change. Aspies who do not like change can have a harder time adjusting. Also, for Aspies with weakness in more abstract language, social misunderstandings can become more common as their peers use more sophisticated language.

Understanding Personal Space

We all have an invisible circle around us and feel uncomfortable when someone we don't invite into the circle comes inside, especially if it is unexpected. Your child has this same circle and may be very adamant about others not getting too close or touching. Even so, he probably doesn't yet understand that other people also feel uncomfortable, and he will often invade someone's personal space.

The concept of personal space is an abstract term and can be different for each person. A general rule for not invading another person's personal space is to stand approximately 3 feet away when talking to someone. To make it easier for your child, institute the "arm's length" rule. He should make sure there is enough room for him to spread his arm straight out between him and the other person. This is more concrete and easier than your child carrying a tape measure and measuring 3 feet when talking to someone.

John was getting into trouble in middle school for "sexual harassment" of the girls. When pressed by his parents, the school administrator finally defined John's "harassment" as "standing too close to the girls and making them feel nervous." Initially, John was sent to the counselor because of this "problem." She tried a typical therapy technique of reversing the roles and having John pretend he was a girl and that the counselor was John. She asked him to tell her to stop walking toward him when he became uncomfortable. John said he understood. However, when they role-played it, John never said stop. The counselor started putting things like "oppositional" in her notes. When later asked directly by someone trained in working with AS youth, John explained it clearly: "I was never uncomfortable, so I never said stop." John was taught the arm's length rule and practiced it, with a closed hand, one-on-one with his speech therapist until he felt comfortable judging the distance by eye in the real world. His referrals for "sexual harassment" stopped after he was taught this simple rule and allowed to practice it with direct and clear feedback.

Aggression

Young children typically use aggressive behavior to get what they want or when they are afraid. They may grab a toy from another child or become angry if they don't get their way. As children mature, they learn these strategies don't work as well as being nice and cooperating with other children. Your child may continue to rely on aggressive strategies because they have worked in the past.

> **The Doctor's Take**
>
> Before reacting to aggressive behavior in your child, try to find out why it is occurring. It could be from sensory issues, anxiety, or frustration in not knowing what to do. Punishing your child will not help him learn what to do the next time. Focus on an alternative behavior that is positive and practice it with your child before they need it next time.

Aggression may be a way of stopping behavior in someone else. Your child knows how to react to certain situations because you, or teachers and therapists, have provided specific steps to take. When these steps don't work, he becomes frustrated and doesn't know what to do and can lash out. For example, suppose a classmate is teasing him in the hallway at school. You have told him when this happens, he should ask the child to stop, walk away, or ask a teacher for help. First he says, "Stop teasing me." But the other child doesn't stop. Your child walks away, but the other child follows him, continuing to tease him. No teacher is around at the moment, and your child has run out of options to choose from. He pushes the other child to make him stop. While the behavior worked in this instance, it can lead to more aggressive behaviors and to your child being identified as the one who is causing the problem. It is therefore very important to proactively teach your child alternative, positive behaviors to aggression.

Total Honesty

Being overly honest doesn't sound like a problem behavioral trait, but for those with AS, honesty sometimes gets them in trouble. The abrupt honesty often sounds rude to others and can result in adverse reactions.

Barry had few friends in school, but Mary played with him every day at recess. One day she came to school in a new dress and asked Barry what he thought. He looked at the dress and said, "I don't like it." Mary was hurt and didn't play with Barry at recess that day. Barry had no idea what he had done wrong; she had asked his opinion, and he gave it.

It is not your child's intention to be mean; he believes that he should tell the truth. He doesn't understand that telling that little white lie is sometimes okay so you don't hurt someone's feelings. To him, it is wrong or immoral to tell a lie. He doesn't understand why someone would be hurt by hearing the truth. Unfortunately, this can make it hard to make and keep friends.

"Honest to a fault" is a saying that could have been coined in response to living with someone with AS. A classic example is when someone takes something from the teacher's desk. The teacher's response is "I don't care who did it, I just want it back." Steve raises his hand and says, "James took it, and it's in his left front pocket." Teach your child there are times that, unless they are asked directly, they should not offer additional information.

Telling the absolute truth can get your child in trouble, too. Madison always felt it was his responsibility to correct people when they were wrong. Madison's family was getting ready to go to a family picnic. When Madison asked what time they were leaving, his father replied, "We will be leaving at 11:00." Shortly after, Madison's mother, who was in the kitchen packing up food, called to her husband and asked what time it was. "It's 10:30; we have half an hour until it is time to go." Madison looked at the clock and said, "Mom, Dad was wrong; it is only 10:24. You have more than half an hour." Madison's father took this the wrong way. He thought Madison was being smart and told him to stop being a smart aleck. Madison was totally confused. He wasn't being a smart aleck. His mother had asked what time it was, and his father had said the wrong time. He assumed his mother wanted to know the right time. He thought he was being helpful.

You can use *social stories* to help your child understand how telling the truth at all times isn't necessarily appropriate. Help him learn to reframe his responses. Rather than telling Mary "I don't like it," he could have said, "It is a nice dress," without inserting what he thought about the dress. In the social story, explain how Mary was looking for affirmation. She believed she looked nice and wanted her friend to agree. Or use social stories to explain how correcting someone, like Madison did with his father, can be seen as saying, "I am better than you." Social stories help explain when it is better to reframe the truth to not hurt someone's feelings or to be quiet rather than correcting someone.

Definition

Social stories were created by Carol Gray and are now used extensively when teaching Aspies. They describe a situation or skill and provide appropriate ways to act. When describing a social situation, the story gives the other person's perspective. It is written in first person in an easy-to-read manner.

Avoiding Being the Rule Enforcer

Your child sees the world in black and white, in right and wrong. He has a need for everything to be right and a need for everything to make sense, and will often point out other people's mistakes or misdeeds.

Paul's teacher had left the room for a minute to speak with another teacher. Before leaving, she said, "No talking while I am in the hallway; everyone keep working on the worksheet I gave you." Of course, when the teacher stepped out in the hallway, several students began talking and giggling. When she returned to the classroom, she said she had heard some talking and asked who was talking. Paul, assuming it was the correct thing to do, spoke up and told the teacher who had been talking. His classmates were angry and called him "tattletale" and "teacher's pet."

During the elementary school years, children learn to show their friendship by sticking up for another person. This sometimes means keeping quiet so a friend doesn't get in trouble. Your child doesn't understand this logic and so, when asked, he will state what happened. His classmates are busy stretching the limits of what they can do, and small infractions of the rules are common, for example, talking when the teacher is out of the room. Because other students feel they can't trust your child, they avoid him or try to bully him into staying quiet.

Teaching your child not to be a tattletale is a complex lesson. On one hand, you want to teach him that he should not lie; on the other hand, he does not need to be the "rule enforcer" for the entire class. You should explain to him that there are certain situations in which it is appropriate and warranted to tell on other children or adults. Some examples of when your child should tell you or his teacher about someone's behavior:

- If someone has touched him in a private area

- If someone has hurt him or is threatening to hurt him

- If another child is in danger

When your child sees someone doing something wrong, ask him to think about the situations in which tattling is okay and see whether any of them fit this situation. If they do not, but he still feels strongly about having to tell a grown-up about what happened, explain that he should do this in private, when classmates or other children are not around. The teacher or other adult can help decide how the situation should be handled.

Asking to Play

There are many unwritten rules of social relationships. We know them, we follow them, and we expect those around us to do so as well. Your child doesn't know or understand these rules. You have taught him certain rules, such as asking whether he wants your attention, but he doesn't take that same general rule and apply it to other situations. Asking other children to play with him or if he can join in their game doesn't come easily to your child. He may sit on the sidelines, waiting for someone to come up to him and feeling lonely if no one does. Or he may jump in a group activity that is already taking place.

Aspie Advice	If your child is having problems joining in games or activities at recess, make a list of children in his class who have played with him. These are the children he can go up to during recess to ask to join in a game. If you don't know who in the class your child should approach, talk to his teacher about asking some of the children to make the first effort or take turns asking your child to join in their game.

Tony was watching some children play tag at recess. No one had asked him to play, but he wanted to join the game. He saw Randy run up, touch Greg, and yell, "Tag, you're it." He did it, too: he ran up to Greg, but instead of touching him, he pushed him and yelled, "You're it." The other kids looked over at Tony and then continued their game, ignoring him. Tony started running around, pushing people, and yelling, "You're it." Randy, Greg, and the other kids saw Tony as intruding on their game, and they told him to go away.

As with other social skills, your child needs to be taught specific steps for entering in conversations, games, or play activities. Paula Gardner, school psychologist for the Southern Columbia Area School District in Catawissa, Pennsylvania, offers parents the following tips for helping their children ask other children to play:

Make sure you have gone over steps to help your child understand cooperative and reciprocal play. In Chapter 11, we provided specific steps for helping your child learn to play in new and creative ways. When your child is comfortable playing with you on the floor, you can ask whether he would like to ask another child to play as well.

Take your child to the playground and talk about how the other children are playing. Depending on your child's age and cognitive development, discuss what the other children are doing and how they interact with one another. Pay attention to how one child asks another to join him on the swings or the monkey bars.

Use social stories to help your child understand what to do. Social stories help your child understand what behavior is expected and how the other children might react.

Outline specific steps for your child. What should he do first? What might happen? Provide concrete ways for him to respond if the other child agrees to play.

Review the rules of social communication. Remind your child that everyone does not want to hear a long monologue about his interest. Even if your child meets someone who shares his interest, the interest may not be to the same degree. Remind your child there is no hitting or pushing and that he should respect the other child's personal space.

> **The Doctor's Take**
>
> Avoid helping out your child too much. Mistakes happen, usually not that serious. It is important for him to learn how to handle failure or mistakes with dignity and how to respond by fixing and avoiding them in the future. Help your child learn how to say "I'm sorry" with conviction and to avoid repeating the mistake. This is one of the essentials to being a good friend that is all too often overlooked in social skills therapy and coaching.

Set up scenarios to help guide your child through the process. You might want to enlist the help of an older child, maybe someone in high school, who is willing to help develop this skill. Set up a time to meet or have the older child come to your home. You can then guide your child through the process of asking to play step by step.

Remember, this process won't happen overnight. It is often a matter of trial and error, finding the right approach for your child. Pay attention to what he is doing and give specific instruction as to what he did right and what he can change the next time. Continue finding ways for your child to practice asking others to play.

Essential Takeaways

- Aspies have a hard time playing with other children because they resist changing the way they play.
- Personal space is an abstract term and may be difficult for your child to understand. Use concrete terms when explaining personal space and other social rules.
- Many Aspies become the "rule enforcer" and alienate other children.
- Aspies need to be taught specific rules for entering conversations or asking to join games and activities.

chapter 13

Social Competence in Preteens and Teens

Places to find friends

Social rules for teens

Taking care of personal appearance

Going on a first date

It is not unusual for your child to be diagnosed with Asperger's syndrome (AS) in the preteen or teen years. As a parent, you wonder why your child still hasn't developed skills for making friends. One mother watched as her 13-year-old son, Joey, sat alone at the end-of-the-year school picnic. Many of the other kids had joined together to start an informal game of kickball, but Joey was sitting by himself at a picnic table. His mother was confused; Joey got along with his classmates, never complaining of teasing, and had even had a few of the other boys over to their house a few times. As she watched him, she felt the pain of loneliness and wanted to reach out to him but knew, at his age, a mom's meddling was worse than being alone. Finally, one of the other boys called to Joey and asked him to join the game, and off he went.

Joey's parents described him as shy, but as she watched him, his mother wondered if that was all that was going on. Joey had always had a hard time making friends, but she didn't see any difference in his ability to join a group from when he was 5 years old. After all, he had spent the entire school year in class with this particular group of children, and many of them had gone through elementary and middle school with him. Shouldn't he feel comfortable enough to join their game?

Joey's mom isn't alone. In the United States, the average age for a diagnosis of AS is between 11 and 12 years old, but many children aren't diagnosed until their teen years or later when parents don't see progress in social skills. In the previous chapters, we explained how parents can work with younger children to develop social skills. In this chapter, we help you understand AS during adolescence and give you ways to continue building social skills.

Making and Keeping Friends

For some Aspies, having friends isn't important, or certainly not as important as parents might think it is. Many Aspies are content spending large chunks of time alone and are happy pursuing their passions, as we explained in Chapter 8. Some find having and being a friend too difficult, especially as friendships become more complex, and make a decision to spend their time alone. But many Aspies crave social interaction and emotional connections with others but simply have no idea how to go about making and keeping friends.

Finding Friends

Before your child can make friends, he has to be around other children his age. For many Aspies, getting along with either younger or older children is easier. Besides school, your teen may spend little or no time with kids his own age. You probably need to take the lead in helping him find places to meet people and help him evaluate the different options to find some that fit his needs and his interests. Following are some of the places to meet others:

When searching for a friend, your child may need to spend time observing his peers, looking for clues about what the other teens are interested in and identifying those who share interests. At home, help prepare some questions to help him stay focused on a conversation before attending a second get-together or club meeting.

School clubs. Contact your child's school and request a list of all clubs and after-school activities. Don't depend on your child bringing the list home or coming home telling you what clubs he wants to join. Be proactive and look through the list, choosing several that match your child's interests. Then go through the list together and pick one to start with.

YMCA or YWCA. These organizations generally have gyms, pools, and classes on a variety of subjects and interests. Because they are much more informal than in school and dedicated to a particular interest, your child might be able to meet peers who share his interests.

Community classes. You probably already know what topics your child is interested in; use his passions to find activities and classes in your area that match or expand his interests. Ideas include music, art, photography, dance, or martial arts. You might want to ask class size and look for small classes in which he won't feel overwhelmed but has the chance to practice social skills in an informal setting where he is sharing information on a topic he cares about.

Churches and places of worship. Start with your own church, and if there is no youth group, talk with your minister and ask about other churches in your area that have youth groups.

Athletics. Individual sports, such as martial arts, swimming, or track and field, give your child the opportunity to feel part of a team or organization but not singled out as "the weak link" on the team. Other individual athletic activities include bike riding, horseback riding, weight training, and skating.

Team sports. Although many Aspies feel uncomfortable with team sports, some want to participate. Help your child understand the rules of the game and where the game is played. Some Aspies have a hard time with team sports because they don't like anyone to lose, and while their teammates are cheering on the team, they are sitting off to themselves, uncomfortable at cheering for the other team to lose. Other Aspies may be perfectionists and have a hard time losing. Remind your teen that it is the effort that he puts into the game that is important and his goal is to have fun, not to win or lose.

Performing arts. Besides local music classes, your child's school or church may have opportunities to join band, chorus, or choir. Many schools also put on one or two plays or shows per year, with opportunities to act or to be part of the stage crew.

Aspie groups. Some high schools have support groups for Aspies, giving your child an opportunity to meet other children in their own area that are "like them" and can help support and encourage one another. If your child's school doesn't have a group, talk with the guidance office about setting one up or look on the internet to find out whether there are outside groups in your area.

> **The Doctor's Take**
>
> Your teen may focus most of his attention on one passion and feel that he doesn't have any other interests, preventing him from meeting new people. Help your teen create an interest inventory, listing different activities and topics he enjoys, such as bike riding, exercise, working on the computer, cooking, animals, sports, reading, watching movies, and playing video games. Help him be specific so he understands that he has many different topics to talk to peers about.

Participating in different activities will give your child the opportunity to meet new people, practice social skills, and learn to interact with a wide variety of different types of people. Be sure to monitor the situation to make sure it is not causing too much stress, that your child is not being teased or bullied, or that his schoolwork is not suffering.

Understanding the Unwritten Rules of Friendship

Now that you have chosen several ways for your preteen or teen to meet other people, he will need to understand that social rules for teens may not necessarily be the same as the social rules he learned for playing with other children during elementary school. To your child, it seems that everyone besides him knows the rules of friendship and understands what it means to be a friend. We often take our understanding of friendship for granted; we just "know" how to be a friend. As an Aspie, your child may need specific explanations of the responsibilities of being a friend—the unwritten rules of friendship. Some examples are:

Be yourself. Some Aspies find it easy to mimic another person, but they often carry it too far, mirroring actions, words, phrases, types of clothes, and mannerisms—essentially hijacking the other person's personality. It is true that people who "fit in" look, sound, and act like they fit in, and your teen can learn about social interactions by observing and adopting some of the common mannerisms, clothing, and speech of other teens. However, he needs to continue to be himself and be accepting of who he is.

Believe in your friends. Because Aspies are notoriously honest and believe that other people say what they mean and mean what they say, it may be hard for them to sort out the gossip and rumors from the truth. Explain that gossip and rumors are common during these years, but that it is important for him to not believe everything he hears about others. If someone is talking about a friend, he should defend his friend and, in private, talk to the friend to find out the entire story.

Actively listen to your friend. Other people like to know that you think what they have to say is important. Being a good listener is an important part of friendship. Eye contact is one way to let a friend know you are paying attention when he talks. If that is difficult for your teen, suggest he explain this to the friend but show other ways he is listening such as asking questions or leaning in toward the other person.

Your friend wants you to be honest but doesn't always want your honest opinion. This is a matter of tact, a way of being honest while being diplomatic. Help your teen understand how to reword responses so they are not offending others. For example, if a friend gets a new haircut and asks, "How do you like it?" your teen needs to know how to reply, even if he thinks it looks terrible. Talk about different ways of rewording responses so he can be honest without offending others.

Pay attention to your friend's moods. Although it is hard for your teen to read facial expressions and body language, he can learn how different things affect his friends. Teach him to be observant and ask questions, and he will eventually be able to see whether his friend is happy, sad, excited, or upset. Learning to respond to different moods shows he is attentive and caring.

Friendships start as acquaintances and deepen through shared interests and experiences; some acquaintances remain someone whom you can talk to but never become friends. There are also different levels of friendships. For example, a teen might talk to the same person every day in science class and consider that person a friend, even though they do not see each other outside of school or share the same level of trust as a close friend. Your teen needs to learn to classify friends and other people he knows into different categories and understand what types of things he can talk about with each category.

Hygiene and Appearance

Throughout this book we have mentioned that many Aspies aren't concerned with their appearance. Because of sensory issues, some find bathing or showering uncomfortable; because they frequently are out of touch with what peers are thinking, they don't worry about fads or trends in clothing. All of this can lead to your teen not only feeling different but looking out of place as well. In Chapter 3, we offered suggestions on how you can use the internet or enlist the help of other teens to find out what is fashionable, and this is just as important for boys.

Brian didn't see the need to shower every day. The strong smell of the soaps and shampoos bothered him, using deodorant irritated his skin, and brushing his hair and his teeth was painful. He avoided these tasks as much as possible, showering only when his parents insisted. His clothes were what he called "comfortable." He preferred nylon basketball shorts and a T-shirt; jeans were tight and made him uncomfortable all day, and button-down shirts took forever to get on in the morning. He frequently grabbed whatever clothes he saw in the morning, even if he had worn the same shorts and shirt for several days. It didn't bother him, and he couldn't understand why his parents made a big deal about him wearing the same clothes more than once.

The Doctor's Take

It is often uncomfortable for non-Aspies to be as blunt as they need to be in order to communicate effectively with an Aspie. Being blunt is often misperceived by many as being rude. However, it is often essential that you be blunt in order to effectively communicate with your Aspie audience. Saying "You stink!" to a non-Aspie might result in a fight or your being ignored. Saying to an Aspie "You smell and need a shower," when true, is being blunt and may result in them taking a shower, where something more subtle or typical might be completely missed.

Other than the obvious health benefits of personal hygiene, your teen's appearance makes a difference in how he is accepted at school and other social functions. Aspies already feel different than their peers because of their way of thinking and processing information. Poor hygiene and dressing differently only adds to their sense of isolation. You can help your teen in a number of ways:

Have your teen accompany you to the pharmacy or grocery store to choose hygiene products. Because of sensory issues, he may have a hard time with strong-smelling soaps, shampoos, and deodorants. Have him smell the different products and choose which ones he prefers. Try different deodorants, such as unscented or aerosol, to find those he finds least irritating. Pick out different flavor toothpastes and different types of toothbrushes, such as electric, battery operated, or soft bristle. Your teen may be more apt to use products he has chosen.

Set up a daily schedule for hygiene, listing all the tasks to be completed. Explain that certain things must be done more than once a day, such as brushing teeth, but showering can be done once per day. Some teens find sensory issues are heightened at certain times of the day, such as early morning or evening, so let him decide whether he showers first thing in the morning or at night before going to bed. Explain that at times, such as after exercise, he will need to shower more than once per day. If he finds showering prickly or painful, let him take a bath instead. Listening to which tasks cause problems and finding solutions will help him better follow the daily schedule.

Choose clothes that are comfortable and blend in with what other teens are wearing. This takes some planning but helps your teen "fit in" at school. Do some research to find out what peers are wearing and have your teen go shopping with you to find clothes that are comfortable and won't attract attention as being too different. T-shirts or soft cotton shirts are usually okay but look for ones without tags. Pants with elastic or drawstring waists might work better than those with snaps and zippers. Slip-ons or shoes with Velcro help and are available in many of today's styles.

Aspie Advice

Have your teen lay out clothes the night before. You can also have your teen lay out clothes for the entire week. You can hang sweater storage units that have five separate areas in your teen's closet and have your teen place one outfit in each section so he is prepared each morning with a clean set of clothing.

Your preteen or teen probably thinks in very linear ways and may not understand all the reasons that hygiene and appearance matter. At 15 years old, Tom changed his clothes each day because his parents told him to but he didn't really see the point. To him, it was a waste, especially if he hadn't spilled anything, or there were no stains on the clothes. He didn't see why he needed to take a shower every morning. Sure, he agreed that he should clean up after exercise, but on days he didn't do much or break a sweat he didn't bother. He didn't worry or even notice other people's appearance and therefore didn't think anyone should care about his.

Your child will follow a daily schedule if he logically sees and understands the reasons. Help by explaining that a neat and clean appearance shows others that he respects himself. His classmates want to know that he respects them, and if he doesn't care about himself they will believe he doesn't care about others.

Further explain to your teen that good hygiene is important to health. Washing his hands before eating or when coming in from outside reduces chances of spreading germs or getting sick. Brushing his teeth is important to oral and overall health, not to mention keeping breath fresh. While the latter might seem less than logical to your teen, others will likely appreciate it. And washing his hair helps keep it healthy and can reduce uncomfortable scalp issues.

In many ways your teen will stand out in a positive way: intelligence, knowledge about a specific topic, honesty, loyalty, and problem-solving abilities, but these will be overlooked if he is ignored or avoided because of his appearance. Let him know that first impressions matter. In order to let classmates get to know him, his appearance shouldn't drive them away. Although the absolute latest fashions aren't necessary, having a neat and clean appearance is, and it matters.

Dating and Relationships

Dating is a big step for a teen with AS, and you probably look forward to this stage with both anticipation and dread. Although "the first date" is a rite of passage, showing your child is growing up, you probably aren't sure whether your child is ready, or how he will manage all the nuances of a first relationship. Even the very beginnings of the relationship are difficult.

Micah, a junior in high school, had several classes with Patty, and they usually walked from one class to the next together. Micah was fascinated with computers and often fixed his classmates' computers whenever they had a problem. Patty was planning on going to college to study programming, so she and Micah had plenty to talk about. While they talked Patty often smiled, touched Micah on the arm, and told him how much she liked talking to him, hinting that she would like to spend more time with him. Another classmate, Rich, commented to Micah that Patty was interested in Micah and wanted him to ask her out. Micah wondered if Patty had told Rich this, but he said "No, I can see it in the way she flirts with you when you walk to class." Micah had no idea what Rich was talking about.

Dating and romantic relationships begin with flirting, and much of flirting is body language: a look, a touch, playful teasing, leaning in toward someone when he is talking. Knowing when someone is interested in you or is flirting with you requires the ability to read behind the words and actions, one of the weaknesses of teens with AS. Micah thought Patty was a friend and even liked her but did not understand the signs that she was interested in developing a relationship.

misc.

Talking on the Phone

As your teen begins dating, talking on the phone becomes important. Use scripts to teach him how to answer the phone, how to leave messages, and how to hold a conversation over the phone rather than in person.

Even beyond the flirting stage, teens with AS don't always know what to do. Tommy was able to ask girls out. He had asked four different girls out, usually by text message, and they had all said yes, but he still hadn't gone on a date. After a girl said she wanted to go out, he had no idea what to do, and the relationship fizzled before it even began. Many teens without AS begin separating from their parents at this time, learning from these new types of relationships on their own. But your teen still needs your help. Your teen, like Micah and Tommy, needs direction and help in navigating romantic relationships.

First Date

Scripts can help your teen by giving him the words to say in different situations. Work together to come up with different ways to ask someone out or to respond if someone else does the asking. By preparing in advance, your teen can be prepared when someone likes him, but keep communication open so that scripts can be changed to match the personality of the specific person your child is interested in.

When your teen is ready to go out on the first date, help him decide what to wear and where to go. We talked about girls with AS in Chapter 3 and discussed some of the areas you need to prepare your daughter for, such as someone taking advantage of her, but boys will benefit from this as well. Some of the concerns with boys occur because of their inability to read emotions in other people. Some will ignore the rules of "taking it slow" and move much too quickly, scaring the girl away, or will talk about their passion throughout the evening, ignoring signs that his date is bored or not interested. Others don't understand the importance of letting a date know he likes her company.

Although you don't want the entire night to be scripted, your teen will need some direction on what to talk about and how to fill in the silences. Some of the areas you want to write scripts for might include:

- What to say when he greets his date
- What questions to ask to show his date he cares about her interests
- How to let a date know she looks nice

- How to let a date know he would like to see her again

- How to end the date

Be sure to talk to your teen about discussing his passions. Even if his date shares an interest in the same passion, have your teen set limits on how long to talk about his special interest and to remember to take turns talking, allowing his date time to talk as well.

Sex

If you haven't talked to your teen about sexuality and sex, he may have formed his opinions of sexuality and how to act based on what he has seen on television, in the movies, or what he has heard about celebrities in the news. Unfortunately, the media doesn't always show an accurate description of how to act in public. Your teen might believe that openly flirting or using sexual innuendos, making sexual advances, or using explicit sexual language is appropriate behavior to show someone he cares. When working on scripts, as we described in the previous section, make sure to include a discussion on what is appropriate and inappropriate language.

> **The Doctor's Take**
>
> Attraction to someone of the same sex is not limited to non-AS teens. Be prepared that romantic interests may be of the opposite sex or the same sex. Either way, your teen needs your support, understanding, and help to foster healthy relationships.

It may be uncomfortable for you to talk about sex and sexuality with your teen, but it is essential—not talking about it will not make it go away or be any less relevant in your teen's life. Not talking about it will only make them less prepared and less knowledgeable about the subject when the time comes. When beginning a discussion, ask your teen direct questions to find out what he already knows and to find out the accuracy of what he knows. Ask about his desires and what he worries about, and talk about normal behavior and how behaviors change as a relationship develops and deepens.

As your teen sees that you are comfortable with the subject (even if you are just pretending) he will be more comfortable and open, coming to you when he has questions or concerns. This helps as you continue your discussions to include responsible sexual behavior and the risks of irre-sponsible behaviors including unwanted pregnancy, sexually transmitted diseases (STDs), and AIDS/HIV. Some Aspies, because of their need for connection, may enter into sexual relationships early. Your conversations need to explain condoms, birth control pills, other forms of contraceptives, and the importance of having an exclusive relationship when building and maintaining trust and as a way to reduce the risk of STDs.

Just as with earlier social relationships, your teen needs specific informa-tion during every step of a romantic relationship. Intense emotions can make him feel overwhelmed, and he may react by acting out or with-drawing. Pay attention to the signs of deep emotional feelings, and most importantly, keep communication open with your teen during this time.

Essential Takeaways

- Helping your child get involved in different types of school and community activities will help him be exposed to and meet friends.
- Aspies have a hard time understanding the unwritten rules of friendships. Explaining what these rules are helps him to fit in with his peers.
- Aspies may not care about their clothes or personal hygiene, so you may need to set specific rules on how often he showers and performs other personal hygiene tasks.
- Teens with AS don't always understand when someone is inter-ested in them romantically.
- As a parent, you will need to communicate about sexual behaviors.

Bullying

The majority of children with Asperger's syndrome (AS) are bullied at some time or another during their childhood. Some Aspies state they are the victim of bullying one or two times per week. In this chapter, we focus on bullying within the school, but this doesn't just happen at school. It also happens in their neighborhood, on sports teams, when participating in after-school activities, and sometimes within the home. All children deserve the right to feel safe at school and to go through their day unafraid.

Types of Bullying

When thinking about the word "bully" many of us imagine pushing, shoving, and name calling, and although these are all examples of bullying, these behaviors are only some of the ways bullies intimidate others. Bullying is usually defined as repeated behavior, such as verbal harassment, physical assault, coercion, or manipulation, with the intention of causing harm or to gain power over another person. The victim of bullying is usually someone who is physically, psychologically, or socially weaker than the bully.

Face-to-Face Bullying

Face-to-face, or direct, bullying frequently happens at school, on the bus, as children are walking back and forth to school, at recess, in the lunchroom, and other areas where there is less teacher supervision. But school isn't the only place your child can be bullied. He might face teasing and aggression in your neighborhood, while playing sports, in after-school clubs and activities, and even in your own home. Some examples of physical bullying behavior include:

- Physical actions, such as pushing, shoving, hitting, punching, kicking, pulling hair, scratching, purposely tripping someone, or stealing lunch or other belongings

- Humiliation through teasing; calling names; criticizing in front of others about disability, dress, culture, race, religion; spreading rumors or gossiping; or pulling a chair out from behind someone to watch him fall

- Manipulation or coercion; for example, pretending to be friends with someone for the purpose of embarrassing him, having someone do something to try to get him into trouble, or telling him if he does something (often something against the rules) they can be friends and then laughing at him

- Social exclusion, such as boycotting a person's party, intimidating peers who are nice or trying to be friends with the victim, or purposely excluding him from games or activities

The Doctor's Take

Aspies see the world in black and white and don't always understand the gray areas. When bullying takes the form of physical abuse, they can recognize the signs, but when mistreatment is more psychological, it isn't that easy. Without the ability to read social cues and understand the difference between good-natured teasing and cruelty, your child may accept abuse from classmates in silence.

Cyberbullying

This type of bullying uses digital media to harass and humiliate another person. Using text messages, social networking sites, blogs, websites, instant messaging, email, and interactive gaming, children are criticized and ostracized. Some examples of cyberbullying include:

- Sending hateful text messages, forwarding inappropriate pictures, or sending criticizing messages about your child to the entire class

- Enlisting the help of classmates to send thousands of text messages to your child's cell phone

- Stealing passwords to social networking sites or emails and changing profile information or posting mean things about other people under your child's name

- Using public blog/websites/message boards to post humiliating or critical things about your child

- Sending pornography to your child through instant messages or texts

- Using foul language or humiliating your child during sessions of interactive gaming, such as using X-Box Live

When your child is faced with this type of bullying, the effects could be even more traumatic than face-to-face bullying. Sometimes cyberbullying is anonymous, which can heighten your child's anxiety because he doesn't know who, from all those he knows, might be the one bullying him. Or an anonymous statement is reinforced by classmates and other children, making your child feel as if everyone is against him. If he is bullied at school, he can arrive home and feel safe and secure, but with cyberbullying, no place is safe. With the widespread use of phones and other devices that surf the Net, the harassment and abuse follow him wherever he goes.

Why Aspies Make Good Bully Targets

Typically, children who are different, don't "fit in," are socially awkward, or are perceived as weak are those who arc bullied. Aspies fit into this category and are often targeted by bullies. Some experts indicate that up to 94 percent of all Aspies are bullied at some time in their lives. As a parent, you can help by being aware of the reasons Aspies are picked on and work with your child to improve skills in these areas.

- Because Aspies are frequently not concerned with physical appearance, fads, trends, popular music, or hairstyles, they stick out as being different than their classmates.

- Aspies are often seen as loners, sitting alone at lunch and not playing with others at recess. Lacking a social network tends to make these children easy targets.

- Your child might make remarks or comments that he sees as the truth but are considered rude, offensive, or insulting by peers.

- Aspies sometimes resist taking showers, brushing teeth, or brushing their hair, causing other children to tease them as dirty or smelly.

- Aspies have poor social skills, saying the wrong thing at the wrong time, answering questions incorrectly in class, or making social blunders.

> **The Doctor's Take**
>
> No one wants their child to be bullied. In addition to addressing the specific bullying, it is very helpful to try to identify what may have triggered your child being singled out; for example, Aspies can sometimes continually correct others or act as the classroom "rule enforcer," which can lead to derision. There isn't always a readily identifiable reason, but if there is, it may be something that you can help your child change in order to minimize the risk of a repeat of the bullying in the future.

Some Aspies are "people pleasers" who dislike any type of conflict; other students can take advantage of your child's willingness to comply with any request. He may also be more willing to accept abuse from other students because negative attention is better than no attention. Although it is important to understand some of the reasons Aspies are targeted by bullies, it is just as important to make sure your child understands that being bullied is not his fault.

Emotional Effects of Being Bullied

In the past, bullying was sometimes seen as a normal part of childhood. Comments such as "boys will be boys" or "it will help him build character" were common. Research over the past decade has shown this isn't the case. Children who are victims of bullying often carry the emotional scars from bullying throughout their lives. The U.S. Department of Justice states that bullying can have lasting effects and result in depression or anxiety disorders that last into adulthood.

Your child might not tell you what is going on, not understanding that he is being mistreated because he can't tell the difference between mild teasing and abuse, or he is unable to effectively communicate what is happening. Unfortunately, when your child is bullied, he may replay the incident in his mind, over and over, sometimes hundreds of times. This means that the emotional devastation is felt over and over, making the feelings of isolation and loneliness that much worse.

Signs of Bullying

If you are worried about whether or not your child is being bullied at school or elsewhere, the first step is to talk with him, asking direct questions about how other children are treating him and letting him know that if something is going on, you are there to help. But Aspies aren't always able to communicate their feelings or frustrations with other behaviors and may be worried about getting other children in trouble. Although the following signs can't tell you definitively if your child is being bullied, if you notice any of these signs, it should raise a red flag for you to look further into how your child is being treated.

- Lost, missing, or damaged possessions
- Coming home from school unusually hungry, as if he hasn't eaten his lunch

- Bruising or other signs of physical injury

- Changes in sleeping patterns, having problems sleeping, waking up several times during the night or sleeping more, or not wanting to wake up

- Complaints of frequent headaches or stomachaches

- Doesn't want to go to school

- Aggression when he wasn't aggressive previously

- School performance slipping

Your child may also show signs of depression or anxiety. In Chapter 4, we listed many of the common symptoms of both of these related disorders.

Working with Your Child's School

Discovering your child is being bullied is emotionally distressing. Your first reaction might be anger; you want to march right over to the bully's house to confront the parents. This is often not a good idea, especially if you do not know the parents and are not sure how they are going to react. Instead, if the bullying is occurring at school or on the way to or from school, start with talking to your child's teacher or principal in private. Explain why you think your child is being bullied and let the teacher and principal know that you are requesting some steps be taken to ensure your child feels safe and secure at school.

Aspie Advice	If your child has a Section 504 or Individualized Educational Plan (IEP), request a meeting so it can be revised to include specific ways of protecting him from bullying.

You can request that an adult aide accompany your child in the hallways and be close by at lunch and recess. Another common accommodation includes having a quiet area at school your child can utilize when feeling stressed; this area can also be used for your child to go to when he is feeling bullied. The school can also set up a "safe zone" that is consistently supervised during lunches and recesses to give all children a place to go when they are feeling intimidated by other students. This can be a certain corner of the lunchroom and playground where extra aides are posted and routinely interact with the children to make sure everyone feels safe.

Enlisting Bystanders

One of the concerns about some anti-bullying campaigns is that they focus on the victim and what the victim can do to avoid being bullied, but neglect to address the bullies themselves. Bullies act aggressive and tease other children in order to be "cool" and to get the attention of other students. They do it for the benefit they receive, and by working to take away that benefit, you take away the motivation to bully. One way to do this is to enlist the help of bystanders.

Bystanders are those students who witness the bullying but do nothing to stop it, because they are either scared of the bully turning on them or because they don't know what to do. Empowering the bystanders helps to neutralize bullies. The first step is to work with teachers and pick out which students have been willing to defend other children. Teachers and other school personnel need to take an active role by showing support and appreciation for compassionate behavior by taking several students aside and complimenting the students on their kind behavior.

If the students are willing, teachers can outline specific steps to take when they see bullying behavior, such as reporting it to the supervising adult, standing up and telling the bully to stop, or being a friend to the student being bullied. Teachers should let the students know that they have their full support and will always take the time to listen and take action on what has been reported and will protect the students from further bullying. By encouraging bystanders to take an active role in stopping bullying behaviors, the bully loses his audience and his reason for bullying.

Anti-Bullying Programs

Many school districts have instituted an "Anti-Bullying Policy," which lists examples of bullying behaviors and explains the resulting disciplinary measures. You should have received a student handbook at the beginning of the school year, and this handbook may include the anti-bullying policy. If it does not, contact the school and ask for a copy of the policy and how the policy is enforced.

Some school districts have a "zero-tolerance" policy, which means the first violent offense is reported to the police. However, teachers and staff often look the other way, excusing inappropriate behavior from athletes or popular students and instead focusing on what the victim did wrong or what the victim should have done differently.

Dr. Dan Olweus is considered a forerunner in bully research and advocated for laws against bullying in schools, first in Norway and Sweden and later in the United States. He developed a bully prevention program that has been instituted in hundreds of schools around the United States and has shown a great deal of success in reducing reports of bullying, vandalism, fights, theft, and truancy. Some of the adaptations in the program include hiring a bullying coordinator; keeping monitors in lunchrooms, restrooms, hallways, and playgrounds; and making sure there are consistent interventions.

When Your Child is Called a Bully

Sometimes, Aspies are seen as the bully, not the victim. Usually this happens not because they want to hurt the other person, but because they are trying hard to fit in. Consider the following examples:

Joshua sat at the lunch table with a few of the rowdy, unruly boys in his class. They often teased one another, and even though Joshua didn't understand the teasing, he tried to fit in and copy what they did. But Joshua didn't realize that this type of teasing needed to stay among friends. When they returned to the classroom, Joshua loudly started teasing other classmates; sometimes his comments were very insulting, but he thought he was being funny.

Ronnie desperately wanted friends. When a group of boys asked him to join them on the playground, he was thrilled. The boys were picking on one of the other boys and told Ronnie to grab the books from him and throw them on the ground. Not wanting to lose his new friends, he did it. In the coming weeks, the boys told Ronnie to do other mean things to kids, and he did it because it was better than being alone again. In the end, Ronnie was the one who got in trouble and was called the bully.

Nicky had a hard time keeping his emotions under control. Whenever he got frustrated or upset, he would start screaming and waving his hands, often hitting whoever was in front of him. Dan thought it was funny to get Nicky mad and then watch him "lose it," especially because Nicky would end up getting in trouble for hitting someone.

> **Aspie Advice**
>
> If your child is bullying other children, talk about how he would feel if someone acted this way toward him, make sure he writes a written apology or apologizes in person, and continue to follow up with your child and the school to make sure the behavior has stopped.

In these examples, the children with AS all were labeled troublemakers or bullies because of their inability to pick up on social cues or because of their need to be included in a group. It could be argued that all of them were actually victims of bullies.

Strategies for Parents

You can help your child to learn and recognize the signs of being bullied and learn ways to manage their own behaviors and attitudes in a number of ways:

- Teach social skills, focusing on what constitutes bullying and what is typical behavior for children the same age as your child.

- Model behavior at home of tolerance of and acceptance of everyone's differences. Discuss the importance of standing up for those who are weaker or can't stand up for themselves.

- List people your child can trust at school to listen and help to find solutions to problems interacting with other students. Let those on your list know that you have listed them as a trusted adult your child can turn to when needed.

- Give your child specific, numbered ways of dealing with verbal and physical abuse; use exact phrases he can say to the other person and phrases to use to explain what happened.

- Talk to your child's teacher about assigning your child a specific responsibility during group activities.

- Work with your child's school to create a lunch table discussion group. This can be a group of children with a similar interest, a book club, or an Aspies group; ask for a table in a quiet area of the cafeteria.

- If your child has been bullied, ask specific questions about who was involved, what happened, what your child's response was, and who else was in the area.

- Ask the school to provide an optional, structured activity during recess time or to set up an area with extra supervision to give students a safe place to play.

- Look for safe activities outside of school for your child to participate in to help develop self-esteem and social skills.

Most of all, remind your child he isn't to blame and that you will work with him to find solutions. If you see signs of depression or anxiety, talk to your child's doctor immediately.

Essential Takeaways

- Bullying can be physical or psychological and can take place in person or through digital media, such as online, text messaging, or interactive gaming.

- Aspies are often targeted by bullies because they are socially awkward or are perceived as weak by their peers.

- Creating a "safe zone" with your child's school can give your child, and other students, a safe place to go during lunch and recess without the fear of being bullied.

- Because of their desire to fit in, some Aspies will follow other students, even if what they are doing is wrong, and get labeled as a troublemaker or bully.

chapter 15

Ongoing Social Skills in Young Adults

Entering the workforce

Important skills for succeeding at work

The question of disclosing AS

Living independently

As your child finishes high school, you might wonder how he is going to manage the next phase of his life. Even if you have made plans and preparations, you still worry about his ability to succeed in college or at work; to navigate the world outside your home.

There are individuals with Asperger's syndrome (AS) in the medical, computer, music, and other industries who go on to have successful careers. Sometimes, symptoms will lessen as your child matures; some adults no longer meet the diagnostic criteria, but language and communication deficits linger. We'll talk more about college in Chapter 19; in this chapter, we focus on work and independent living, although many of the skills discussed in this chapter, such as when and how to disclose a diagnosis, can help in all adult situations.

Asperger's Syndrome at Work

After high school, your child might opt to enter the workforce full time or attend college part time and work part time. He may need guidance exploring different careers, finding one that incorporates his passions. Parents can also help develop new skills, such as interviewing, working with supervisors, and getting along with co-workers.

Vocational and Interest Assessments

Most experts say that one of the keys to success for Aspies in the workplace is finding a job he relates to, something that stimulates his interests and incorporates his passion. Many Aspies work with a high school guidance counselor or psychologist to complete career and vocational assessments to identify their unique interests and talents.

MISC.

Finding Employment Based on Passions

Tom's passion was anything that related to Ford. When it came time for a job, his combination of precision about keeping things orderly, passion about Ford, excellent memory, and reliability made working at a Ford dealership an obvious choice. A position in the parts department came open, and it was a match made in Heaven. The owner realized what an asset Tom was one day when the computers were down, and Tom still found every part needed by the maintenance department.

A career assessment is a test, or a series of evaluations, that help determine what types of jobs most closely match your child's personality, knowledge, skills, and interests. The results of the test should be used to spur discussions about different types of careers and jobs he is suited for. While he may not find the "perfect" job through the assessment, it can provide ideas he hasn't yet thought about. These tests also offer information on weaknesses, giving him ideas on areas to increase knowledge and skills through noncollege courses, self-study, or online classes to make him more employable.

Mastering the Job Interview

Getting through a job interview is hard. Much of the interview is based not just on how well your child can do the job but on personality. The interviewer wants to know whether he is a "team player" or whether he only works well when working alone. He wants to know whether he can take direction, follow instructions, and get along with co-workers. In other words, he wants to know whether your child is a good fit for his company. Some of the social difficulties, such as lack of eye contact, cause problems in a job interview. Role-playing and practicing interviews helps, but before you begin, go over some of the basics of interviewing:

Practice deep breathing. When feeling overwhelmed or stressed, take a deep breath; remind yourself you can do this.

Remember first impressions count. Aspies don't understand the "sense" of first impression, believing you should judge someone on what is inside and not judge based on appearances, so this concept might be difficult. In this instance, how he greets the interviewer matters.

Dress for the job. The general rule of thumb is to dress "one level up." That means if you are going for a job that requires business casual dress, you should dress professionally; if the job is more of a jeans and t-shirt type of atmosphere, dress slacks and a casual buttoned shirt are appropriate.

> **Aspie Advice**
>
> Interviewers pay attention to body language. Have your child practice sitting still, with his hands in his lap, using good posture and leaning forward when someone is talking to show interest. If he can't look someone in the eye, have him look right below the eye or at the person's ear; looking in the general direction makes someone believe you are looking him in the eye.

Help your child understand his skills, talents, and strengths so he can talk about them. Remind him to answer questions briefly, without rambling, to show confidence in his abilities. Books and websites on interviewing offer many standard interview questions you can practice. Be careful, though, as your child can be prepared for these questions but then be thrown off if the questions are different. Try to ask questions in different ways so your child can adapt his answer based on the question.

Community colleges, continuing adult education, Goodwill, the YMCA, or employment agencies frequently offer job interviewing classes. This gives your child the opportunity to learn about interviewing from people in the community that are, or have been, interviewers. Their feedback can be an essential part of mastering interviewing skills.

Managing Asperger's Syndrome on the Job

After your child lands a job, the next step is to keep the job. Although much of this will be based on your child's ability to do the job, there are some social areas companies take into consideration as well:

Good work habits. Does he show up on time? Does he go to work every day or call in sick too often? Companies want to know your child is reliable and is at work, on time, each day. While this is often not a problem for Aspies as they like structure and following rules, the stress of a new job can be overwhelming. Talk about the importance of allowing enough time in the morning to get through traffic and using personal days sparingly or not at all during the first few months at a job.

Talking professionally. Even if your child's new job is in a relaxed atmosphere, there are unwritten rules for interacting with co-workers. Your child should not use obscene, foul, or offensive language in the workplace. Supervisors will watch to see whether he is polite and respectful of co-workers, such as using "please" and "thank you," and talking to co-workers as equals (even if he is more knowledgeable about the topic).

Changing attitudes based on who he is talking to. Many times Aspies have a hard time adjusting their attitude. They adopt a single approach toward everyone, not understanding how to treat different people differently; but managers look for a submissive attitude toward supervisors, a friendly and cooperative attitude toward co-workers, and a helpful, fair, and kind attitude toward subordinates. You may need to role-play different types of interactions with your child as he learns about different personal interactions in the workplace.

Working independently and as part of a team. Another possible area of contention for Aspies is working within a group. Aspies are often solitary people, preferring jobs where they work independently and are responsible for their own work. But frequently jobs require working with co-workers to complete a project. Explain that there may be times he needs to use ideas and suggestions from others and incorporate those into his own work.

Handling conflicts. No matter how well your child seems to fit into a work environment, there are times when conflict with co-workers will appear. Prepare for these disagreements and work on a plan of action your child can take when he and a co-worker have a different opinion so it doesn't escalate into a more serious situation. This plan can be based on how he handled previous conflicts with classmates or siblings.

If your child is having trouble adapting to a work environment, a *life coach* or mentor could help. Mentors can be found in the business community. Use resources such as AS community groups, support groups, community business groups, and AS organizations and ask whether they know of any mentors in your area. Someone who has AS and has learned to navigate the social difficulties of the workplace can be a sounding board, answer questions, provide encouragement, and give your child advice on how to handle specific situations without him fearing retaliation.

> **Definition**
>
> A **life coach** works with individuals based on specific needs. They can help with organization, social skills, or conflict resolution. Life coaches usually meet or talk with clients on a weekly basis, review how the week went, and set goals for the coming week. Life coaches are not therapists or counselors but work on practical living skills.

Disclosing AS

Whether your child heads off to college or starts a job, he will need to decide whether or not to disclose his AS diagnosis with professors, bosses, co-workers, and fellow students. This is a personal decision; sometimes it helps others understand, while at other times it makes life more difficult. Disclosing is important and necessary if he is asking for accommodations, but might also invite discrimination if others know about the disability. Some people may not understand what having AS means and treat him as if he is stupid or incapable of thinking for himself, creating conflict.

Disclosure often depends on his relationship with that person. Going over different types of relationships and how much to disclose within each helps:

Bosses and college professors. If your child is asking for accommodations either at work or in college, he needs to tell them why. Before disclosing, he needs to know exactly what accommodations he is asking for and why he feels these will help him perform better. When talking to either a college professor or a boss, your child should state his diagnosis and list accommodations. He should not be required to provide additional information.

Acquaintances. Generally, acquaintances don't need to know about your child's diagnosis. The relationship is not deep enough or significant enough for him to feel he needs to share this information.

Roommates, co-workers. Whether or not your child lets roommates or co-workers know about his diagnosis should be based on what he expects to accomplish from disclosing this information. He may want to use the diagnosis to explain certain behaviors and help those he deals with on a daily basis better understand his actions (or inactions). Remember, if your child doesn't want everyone to know about his diagnosis, he will need to be sure he can trust those that he does choose to tell.

Friends. During high school your child decided whether to let friends know that he has AS. This decision was based on trust and a commitment to care about one another and share personal information, so he should already have decided whether he feels comfortable talking about his diagnosis. But sometimes Aspies have a hard time distinguishing between friends and acquaintances and disclose information to people who are not his friends. Create a checklist of important qualities in a friend to help your child determine whether someone is a friend or an acquaintance. Remind your child he has the right to not answer personal questions.

The Doctor's Take

Sometimes the results of disclosure aren't felt until later, as the friend tries to find additional information or understand what a diagnosis of AS means. Often such friends develop a better understanding and caring attitude, and the friendship deepens. Other times disclosure is offered to someone who uses the information against him in a limiting attitude, believing "Oh, he can't do that, he has AS."

Disclosure is tricky; your child may get the desired response, or someone could look at him in total confusion, asking questions or wondering how someone who functions so well could have a disability. Some may feel he is using this as an excuse for poor social skills or as a way to not bother trying. As your child practices disclosure, he will learn how to answer questions and hopefully, from the disclosures that didn't work out so well, will accept there are times not to disclose.

Living Arrangements

Living in a dormitory at college, getting an apartment, having roommates, living alone, or staying in the safe and secure bedroom he has always lived in—what is best? There is no single answer to this question. Your child is unique, his symptoms are unique, and he has learned to cope with symptoms in his own way. There are certain advantages and disadvantages to all the options, and much will depend on his abilities and desires. When making such a major decision, keep in mind that no decision is forever. If you make a wrong choice, or if the choice you make doesn't work out, it can be undone, and you can work on a new plan.

Living at Home

Your relationship with your child changes when he graduates from high school. Whether he is starting college classes, beginning a full-time job, or doing a combination of classes and work, he wants you to see him as more grown up and mature. For example, if you set curfews for what time he needs to be home at night, he may no longer see these as necessary, believing he is responsible for his own life. Help him understand that no matter who it is, when living with others, he will have to have certain rules in place to make those living arrangements work. For example, curfews may be more lenient, but if he is going to be out past a certain time, he needs to call home. No matter how difficult it is, as a parent, you will need to let him make choices and face the consequences of those decisions—good and bad.

Before conflicts arise, set down some revised house rules. There are probably some rules that are non-negotiable, for example, no drugs in the house, no late-night parties, or no romantic partners spending the night in his room. These rules are similar to those for any young adult, but with an Aspie, rules should be specific and not open to interpretation to avoid any future misunderstandings. Following are some of the areas you want to think about when creating your house rules:

Rent. Will your child pay rent, how much will he pay, and when is it due? What will the rent cover—food, shelter, utilities? If it doesn't cover food, is your child expected to buy his own groceries? Will he have a separate refrigerator? What happens when rent is late? Will he have a room that is his alone? What type of privacy can he expect? If he isn't paying rent, is there work around the house he is expected to do in return for room and board?

Chores. What household chores will your child be responsible for? Is he responsible for doing his own laundry? Is he expected to clean up any dishes he uses? Are there additional chores that must be done? When do they need to be done? What happens when he doesn't complete them?

Lifestyle. If your child has friends, what time do they need to be out of the house? Is it different on weekdays than weekends? Will friends be able to spend the night? Is he allowed romantic partners overnight? What are your rules about smoking and alcohol? What is expected of him? Does he need to work a certain number of hours? Go to school?

Working through these issues in the beginning saves you and your child a lot of conflict later. Some parents find it easier to write a contract or lease with everything included so there are no questions later.

Aspie Advice

Respecting your young adult means you should not dictate how he dresses or wears his hair, where he chooses to work or go to school, where he goes after work and on the weekends, or what he eats. These need to be his decisions. Keep in mind, however, that each child is different, and some will need more guidance and assistance in making adult decisions than others.

Your behavior toward your child also needs to change at this time. He is no longer a child; he is an adult, and even though he is still living in your house, you need to respect that he has grown up. You want to be available for advice and continue communicating with him, but you also need to step back and allow him to be in charge of his own life. As difficult as it is to let go, he will never learn to take care of himself if you are hovering over and making decisions for him.

Supported Living

Supported living offers a compromise if you don't believe your child is ready to live on his own, but he is ready to move out and take control of his life. In supported living situations, your child decides where he lives and signs his own lease but receives assistance in areas in which he is struggling. For example, providers help in budgeting, social skills training, or other areas while allowing him to make decisions about his own life.

The process starts with a provider identifying obstacles to living independently by talking with you and your child. Once this initial evaluation is complete, the service provider creates a plan that includes listing services your child will receive based on his unique needs. One of the myths about supported living services is that the goal is to eventually discontinue services, but this is not necessarily true. Some Aspies may find as they learn to take care of themselves some services are no longer needed, and those may be discontinued. However, other services can continue indefinitely.

Some of the services provided may include:

- Helping with selecting and moving into a home

- Choosing roommates

- Purchasing furniture and household items

- Assistance with daily living activities, such as food shopping, menus, food preparation, cleaning, and laundry

- Providing help with budgeting and managing finances

- Companion services

<table>
<tr><td>The Doctor's Take</td><td>Supported living arrangements allow independence while providing support, even in unforeseen circumstances. The most functional that I've seen in the community involved a duplex arrangement with three young men with Asperger's living as roommates on one side and their support couple living on the other side. One time, a scammer rang their doorbell. This person had already hit the support couple's door, and they were on their way over to the young men's side of the duplex to help them deal with this unusual situation.</td></tr>
</table>

When no supported living services are available, family members or friends can provide these types of services, but this can become time consuming and expensive. The goal of these services is to have your child live in a safe, stable home where he is responsible for his own choices in life.

Independent Living

Your child, now a young adult, might want to move out and live in his own apartment and make his own decisions about his life. As a parent, you might be scared he is not ready and want him to remain at home, where you can continue to support him. Remember, many adults with AS live on their own and manage their daily lives, on their terms. This is what you have been preparing him for, and you can continue to support and encourage him to work toward his dreams.

Help him by creating a budget based on his income. Work together to list all his expenses and determine how much he can afford to pay for rent. If he needs help, show him how to look for apartments in the newspaper or on the internet. He may want to go see the different apartments without you, taking his first steps toward independence.

You might also want to go over the skills needed to live on his own and spend time going over things such as how to go food shopping, cooking simple and nutritious meals, buying household items, and paying bills. Talk about the pros and cons of having a roommate—on one hand a roommate helps to reduce the cost of living on his own, but on the other hand, if he prefers to live alone, he may have a hard time tolerating different cleaning habits, work and sleep schedules, preferences to noise levels, and personal behaviors.

Essential Takeaways

- A career or vocational assessment can help your young adult see what types of jobs would be a good match for his skills and interests.

- Disclosing AS is a personal decision and is often based on your child's relationship with the person.

- Whether your child lives on his own or in a supported living situation, you need to respect his right to make decisions about his life.

- Supported living arrangements offer independence within a structured, supportive environment.

Educational Considerations

In Part 5, we begin with services to help even the youngest Aspies and continue through with information and strategies up to college. Educational services for children with AS can begin before the age of 3, with Early Intervention (EI) services that offer different types of therapies to help prepare your child for school.

From elementary school through high school, you, as the parent, must work with teachers and educational professionals to find the right services and accommodations for your child. We guide you through the process, explaining how to request services and monitor your child's progress and give plenty of examples of accommodations for the different stages of your child's education.

Accommodations are also available in college, and we explain what is involved in requesting services and how you, as the parent, can help prepare and support your child during the first year of college.

Our final chapter in this part is meant to be used with your child. We offer specific strategies you can use to teach your child how to take notes and specific ways to use to-do lists to stay organized. For social skills practice, you can work together with your teen using strategies such as role-playing, scripts, and video monitoring.

Requesting Services

Whether your child is a toddler or in high school, he may benefit from receiving services or accommodations to help improve social skills or learn ways to cope with symptoms of Asperger's syndrome (AS). In this chapter, we will review what types of services are available as well as how to request services.

Early Intervention

Early Intervention (EI) services are state-run government programs for children between the ages of 0 to 3 years old that are funded in part through Medicaid. The purpose of EI is to identify and offer services to young children to better prepare them for their school years. In the next section, we discuss some of the more common services offered through EI. Most of these services are available to parents through community-based programs, such as the YMCA, or by contacting medical professionals privately. However, if your child is eligible for EI services, your county and state will coordinate all services and make sure your child receives all necessary interventions.

There is no doubt that EI services work for children on the autism spectrum. A study completed at the University of Washington in 2009 followed toddlers diagnosed with autism for five years. Some of the children were as young as 18 months at the beginning of the study. At the end of the study it was apparent that EI works. Children receiving intensive EI services had significant improvement in IQ and the ability to adapt their behaviors to their environment as compared to children receiving community-based services.

These services are not used for children with AS as often as those with autism, not because services are not appropriate or necessary, but because children with AS are not usually diagnosed before school age. Often children with AS who receive EI services get them for related issues, such as low muscle tone or sensory or coordination issues. As doctors become more aware of early warning signs of AS and can recognize and diagnose AS in the toddler years, EI services will become more relevant for Aspies. You can ask your pediatrician about who to contact for such services and whether they think your child might benefit from receiving them.

Services Included in Early Intervention

Because families using EI services do not need to pay for them, children from low-income households have access to intensive, customized services. EI begins with an assessment of the child's current developmental level and strengths in several different areas, including language, cognitive skills, social skills, and motor skills. After the assessment is complete, a customized program is developed with your input. Services can be provided in your home, in a day care, or in early childhood centers and vary widely from state to state.

EI services use *evidence-based treatments* (*EBTs*) to address your child's developmental needs and to help you learn how to take care of him.

definition

Evidence-based treatments (EBTs) are those that have been proven to work through rigorous research, such as random, double-blind studies or the collection and interpretation of data from patients, doctors, and research. Using EBTs helps eliminate unsound or risky medical practices and protect patients. Ask medical and service providers to share information on why a treatment meets EBT standards.

Areas addressed in EI services are:

- Physical development, including motor skills, vision, and hearing

- Occupational therapy

- Cognitive development

- Communication development

- Social and emotional development

- Psychological services

- Special instruction

- Speech and language pathology

- Vision services

- Adaptive development

- Nutrition services

Services are frequently required to be provided in your home by trained therapists. If services are given outside your home, such as at a child development center, your county will usually provide transportation to and from the center. Your child may also be provided with health services if he needs health care in order to benefit from the other services. As a parent, you are included in all decisions regarding services, and regular meetings are held at a time and place that is convenient for you.

Requesting Early Intervention Services

Often, a medical professional refers your child to the EI program because, during regular check-ups, he has noticed your child is not meeting certain developmental milestones and believes he has a developmental delay. As a parent, if you suspect that your child might need support, you can also contact your county health service and refer your child for EI. When a doctor refers your child, he lists a diagnosis on the request for services. If your child does not have a specific diagnosis, he will be given an evaluation to determine whether he is eligible for services.

After a referral is made, you are contacted by someone from your local EI office (EIO) who provides you with information on what your rights are, explains how your child will be evaluated, arranges for the evaluation and transportation to and from the evaluation if you need it, and makes sure you understand the process.

If your child is evaluated and found to be eligible for services, someone from the EIO will meet with you to explain what happens next. Normally what's next is a meeting with you, your EI coordinator, and members of the evaluation team. You are able to bring people with you to the meeting, such as family, friends, or an advocate. During the meeting, the evaluation team may suggest specific interventions to help your child. They may also ask what support you need and what help you think your child needs.

Aspie Advice	Stay involved in your child's treatment. When you are involved in your child's therapies, it increases his ability to improve. Studies have shown that when parents are not involved, therapy takes longer, and children need to work harder to benefit from the treatment.

After all information is reviewed, the team, with you included, will set goals for your child and work out strategies, activities, and services to help him reach those goals. The team will also list timelines for measuring whether goals have been met and review his progress. You will be asked whether or not you agree with services being offered. If you do not agree, he will not be able to receive the services, but you can request a mediator to help work with both you and the EI team to come to some agreement.

After you have created a plan of action and decided which services will best benefit your child, someone from the EIO will be responsible for over-seeing and implementing the plan and coordinating the services. You can be present during the therapy sessions and ask the providers to teach you exercises and skills so you can work with your child in between sessions. It is important for you to learn as much as you can about how the therapies that help your child are implemented. By knowing more about how the therapies are done, you can supplement the limited time the therapists have by working with your child in as effective a way as possible when he is not in therapy. You will also be a more effective partner with the therapists in updating and designing your child's course of treatment as a result.

Your child's progress will be reviewed on a regular basis. During these meetings, services will be looked at to see whether they are still relevant or whether it would be more beneficial to change to different services. If you believe your child is not making progress or for any reason would like services reviewed, you can request a meeting to do so.

As your child nears the time when EI services are no longer possible, your contact at the EIO will help explain what types of resources are available and help to plan for him continuing to receive services under different providers. Some children won't need any further services; some families will use private early education programs; and some will continue to receive services through their county or public school district. If your child graduates from therapy because he has mastered the skills, then no referral is needed, which is terrific. If he continues to require therapy after his third birthday, then he can be referred to the local public school district for services. Medicaid funding stops going to EI services at the third birthday and is instead directed into the local school system through the state department of education from the federal government. It is important that you make contact with the public schools at least three months before your child turns 3 in order to give them time to review your child's needs, possibly evaluate him, and have meetings in order to determine eligibility and develop services.

When Your Child Reaches School Age

Within the public school system, your child may be eligible for services and accommodations based on the severity of his symptoms and whether those symptoms interfere with his ability to learn. Many parents mistakenly believe that public school services start at kindergarten; however, in most instances eligibility for services begins on the child's third birthday. The Individuals with Disabilities Education Act (IDEA) mandates that school districts find and identify students who have disabilities, whether physical, mental, or emotional, that interfere with their ability to learn and provide services and accommodations to them. While autism is listed as an eligible condition under this law, AS is not but can be included as "autistic" or "other health impaired" or your child may have a learning disability, such as written expression disorder, which will qualify him for services.

If you believe your child requires special services or accommodations, the first step is to make a written request for an evaluation. In this request you should outline what behaviors you are seeing and how these behaviors are causing problems; your letter should be dated, and you should keep a copy for your records. Your child's teacher can also request an evaluation; if this happens, you will receive information about the evaluation as well as a consent form that must be signed. Although a teacher can request an evaluation, the school cannot perform an evaluation without your consent. Depending on the outcome of the evaluation, your child may be eligible for an *Individualized Educational Plan* (*IEP*) or for accommodations under Section 504.

Definition

The **Individualized Educational Plan (IEP)** is a legal document that provides detailed, written plans for meeting the unique educational needs of your child.

It is very important to know that a diagnosis does not automatically make a child eligible for special education services, nor is a diagnosis typically a requirement for eligibility. School staff and the parents as a team consider all relevant information and using educational laws and regulations determine whether a child meets eligibility criteria for special education services.

If you disagree with the conclusions or content of any of the evaluation reports that the school provides, you have recourse under IDEA. You do not have to accept the evaluations conducted by the school staff if you disagree with them, and you may not have to pay for your own evaluations. Under IDEA and the state regulations that come from this federal law, you, as a parent, have a right to have a private evaluation of your child at public expense under certain circumstances—this is called an Independent Educational Evaluation (IEE). The rules on how these are accessed vary from state to state, but you should be provided with a written copy of your "Parent's Rights" under IDEA, which includes IEEs.

Individualized Educational Plans

If your child is found eligible for services under IDEA, the school creates an IEP team that meets on a regular basis to discuss services and accommodations your child needs. As a parent, you are an important part of this team; other people on the team include:

- At least one regular education teacher

- A special education teacher

- A representative of the school district—often a school administrator, such as a principal

- Your child's guidance counselor or someone who is responsible for implementing services and accommodations

- A school psychologist, speech-language pathologist, or someone who is able to interpret the evaluation

- Other school personnel who have experience or knowledge of your child

MISC.

Time Limits

Your school district must complete an evaluation within 60 days of your formal request for an evaluation. A meeting is scheduled within 30 days of the completed evaluation to discuss the results, and you must receive notice of this meeting at least 10 days before the meeting. If your child is deemed eligible for services, the IEP team creates a plan consisting of services and accommodations necessary for your child's education. When a plan has been agreed on, services must be implemented within 10 days.

You are able to invite others to attend meetings with you, such as an educational advocate, professionals who have worked with your child, family members, or friends. These people can attend meetings to provide moral support, to help you understand the process, or to offer advice and negotiate with the school district. Your child is also able to attend these meetings and, as he enters middle school and high school, it is often beneficial as he learns valuable self-advocacy skills. Some school systems have in-house "parent mentors," who are parents of special education students and whose sole job is helping parents navigate the special education maze. Ask your school district's special education department if they have a "parent mentor."

Every IEP is different because every child is different. The educational team should take into consideration your child's unique needs, finding strategies that build on his strengths and improve his weaknesses. IEP meetings can often get sidetracked, focusing on areas your child needs help without addressing ways to build on strengths, but effective plans include both.

An IEP includes basic information about your child, such as contact information, date of birth, current grade, a list of the special considerations (speech and language impairments, communication issues), a summary of his strengths (including listing his passions), and a summary of his needs. Agreed-upon goals are listed, with objectives for reaching the goals. Each goal should be specific with information on how and when measurement should happen. An example of an IEP goal would be:

Goal—Brenda will use a computer to submit homework to teachers by the end of the first quarter.

Objectives

- Brenda will learn the functions of the computer.
- Brenda will learn how to complete and save homework assignments on the computer.
- Brenda will set up an email account.
- Brenda will learn how to send, receive, and read emails.
- Brenda will learn how to attach a file to an email.
- Brenda will send assignments to teachers.

A cornerstone of IDEA regulations is that all goals must be objectively measureable. Each goal should have clear, clean definitions to determine whether it has been achieved or not. It is no longer acceptable for the criteria to be simply "teacher observation" or "teacher opinion." Each step in this goal should have a time limit or specific dates to review goals so that parents and teachers can monitor progress. Your child's IEP is reviewed by the entire team on an annual basis to decide whether accommodations are still needed and to determine whether new services or accommodations should be included. Goals will be reviewed and adjusted based on your child's progress. In addition to the annual review, as a parent, you can request a review at any time during the school year.

Section 504

Section 504 is a civil rights law that prohibits discrimination against individuals with disabilities. Any institution receiving federal funds must comply with Section 504. Any person with a physical or mental impairment that substantially limits one or more major life activity, such as learning, is qualified. When your child does not qualify for special education services, he could still qualify for accommodations under this law, which is more flexible than IDEA. Accommodations set up under Section 504 are legally binding, just as an IEP is.

Schools may encourage you to apply for accommodations under Section 504 because it can be beneficial to both the student and the school. Section 504 agreements are quicker and do not label a child as "special education" as IEPs frequently do. However, more extensive services, protections, and accommodations are available under an IEP.

IEP vs. Section 504

Misc.

Some parents believe that a child who is eligible for services under IDEA must automatically be placed into special education classes and those eligible for services under Section 504 remain in regular classrooms, but this is not true. Children should be placed in the least restrictive environment, which means that if he can succeed in a regular education class with some modifications and accommodations, he should remain in a general education class.

Section 504 guarantees your child will not be discriminated against because of his disability. Many people consider this a way of "leveling the playing field." For example, your child may need extra time to process written text during test taking. A common accommodation might be to have extra time to complete the test, thereby allowing him the same opportunity to pass the test as the other students. Section 504 gives your child access to the same level of education as others his age are receiving, but it does not guarantee that your child will succeed.

Solving Disagreements with the School

There may be times you can't come to an agreement with your school district, either because your child is found ineligible for services, or you don't believe the school is providing all the services you feel are appropriate. At your original meeting, whether through IDEA or Section 504, you should have received a packet of information that outlines the steps to take when you and the school disagree.

Steps to Take

If, at any time, you disagree with the school district regarding your child's IEP, you can request an impartial due process hearing; just as you requested the initial evaluation, this must be in writing. The officer who conducts the hearing is an employee of your state department of education, or an independent court under your state law, not your child's school district. This hearing should take place within 30 days of your written request. The hearing officer hears both sides and provides you ample time to explain why you do not agree with the school's decision. He must provide his decision within 45 days of your original request for the hearing.

In some instances it may be necessary for you to hire an attorney in order to adequately present your case during the due process hearing. If you need an attorney, it is important to know that there are attorneys who specialize in special education law. Although any attorney can represent people in the due process hearing, it may be best to seek the support of someone versed in both federal special education law and your state's special education regulations specifically.

Fighting for Your Child's Rights

MISC.

It is sometimes necessary for parents to continue fighting to make sure their child receives services. In the case of the Deal family, the administrative hearing found the school to be "appalling," "evasive," "closed minded," "combative," and "untruthful," in failing to provide services to a 7-year-old with autism. The school appealed, and the Federal District Court ruled in favor of the school district. The parents appealed this decision, and the Federal Appellate Court upheld the original findings in favor of the parents.

Either you or the school district has the right to appeal this decision. Appeals of due process hearings are sent to the Federal District Court for initial review and from there to the Federal Circuit Court of Appeals. States vary in how they handle the due process hearing itself with some, like Georgia, having a separate court to hold a hearing with a black-robed judge, and so on, while other states have lawyers who hold the hearings less formally, like Alabama. There may be filing restrictions, such as the date you must file by, in these courts, and if you have not yet hired an attorney, it is probably beneficial at this point. These types of drawn-out battles with a school district are draining, emotionally and financially, for parents but can end up setting precedents for your child as well as future students.

Being Your Child's Advocate

Throughout your child's school years, you spend time talking to teachers and other school personnel about his needs and, at times, fighting for his right to receive those services as well as fighting for specific services you believe he needs. The following tips can help you:

Keep accurate records. Use a binder to hold all of your child's educational papers, including report cards, evaluations, and summaries of meetings and conversations with teachers and other school personnel.

Write down questions or concerns as you think of them. Too often, you have specific questions but once you reach a teacher, you forget what you wanted to ask. Writing down questions and summarizing a teacher's responses helps assure you all your questions and concerns are addressed.

Be prepared when meeting with teachers and school personnel. Besides having questions and concerns written down, make copies of reports or evaluations to share with teachers. Show examples of schoolwork to explain your point of view. Holding back information never helps; you are asking teachers to form or share your opinion based on partial information.

Bring an advocate, family member, or friend if you are feeling overwhelmed. You should be allowed to have someone in all meetings with you, if only for moral support; this person can take notes or share additional information about your child. You may have a right to record your meetings. The laws and rules vary from state to state on whether you have to disclose that you are recording, so it is best to let people know that you are doing so.

Speak up when you don't understand something. Often, people within a specific industry use terminology specific to that industry. Teachers and school personnel might say things like "inclusion" that they fully understand but you do not. Ask questions so you can make informed decisions about your child's education. People who are genuinely trying to be helpful always want those present to understand what is being said. Remember there is no "stupid question."

Share knowledge about your child. As his parent, you are the expert on your child—no one knows him as well as you. If you understand he is either a visual or auditory learner, let his teachers know this. If you understand certain behaviors signal an upcoming meltdown, share this information. Never assume that because they are professionals, they should know all of this. They have many children to work with, and the more information you can supply about your child, the better they can help.

The Doctor's Take

Organization and detailed notes are essential. I recommend that parents invest in a scanner, if possible, and scan *all* documents relating to their child's needs, services, evaluations, treatments, and performance. Having documents in Adobe PDF format makes them easy to access and share with others. If you use notebooks, separate the documents based on the type of records (for example, medical, psychological, speech, OT, school, and so on) and organize them chronologically with the newest at the end.

Working with an Educational Advocate

As a parent, you might decide to work with an educational advocate to help as an intermediary during school meetings. Advocates sometimes work with you by meeting with you and your child and giving suggestions, identifying obstacles to school success, and creating a plan of action that you can use during school meetings. An advocate can also attend meetings with you and negotiate with the school district or help to hold the school accountable for implementing services.

Following are some of the reasons you might choose to work with an advocate:

- Your child's school has denied a request for modifications or accommodations or is denying a specific service you feel would be beneficial for your child.

- You don't have the time or resources to be your child's advocate.

- You don't have the knowledge or self-confidence to be your child's advocate.

- You have been working with the school district and have come up with accommodations, but your child doesn't seem to be making progress.

Although many times, working with an advocate is helpful, your school can see requesting an advocate as a confrontational move. If you have had a good relationship and suddenly choose to hire an advocate, they can become defensive and less willing to cooperate. No matter what, hiring an advocate or an attorney is a personal decision and should be made on the basis of whether it is in the best interest of your child.

In most states, if you decide to take an attorney with you to any IEP meeting or IDEA event, you have an obligation to inform the school district ahead of time because they have a right to legal representation being present, too. Under most state regulations, you are not obligated to inform the district if you are taking anyone else, other than an attorney, with you to such meetings.

Essential Takeaways

- Early Intervention services are effective in improving the ability to adapt behaviors to environment in young children.

- Children with AS may be eligible for services and accommodations in school under the Individuals with Disabilities Education Act.

- Section 504 is a civil rights law that can provide accommodations or modifications for children not meeting eligibility for an IEP.

- During your child's school years, you need to be an advocate for him.

chapter 17

Individualized Help for Your Child

> Ideas for classroom accommodations
>
> Sample goal in an IEP
>
> Homework strategies
>
> Keeping in touch with teachers

Individualized Educational Plans (IEPs) or Section 504 agreements are based on your child's individual needs; no two are alike. As explained in Chapter 16, you and a team of educational professionals work together to determine what accommodations and modifications your child would benefit from during school. In this chapter, we provide examples of some common class-room accommodations and services to help your child in school as well as ways to continue working with him at home.

Examples of Special Services in School

As your child advances in school and develops emotional maturity, his needs change. Frequently, symptoms of Asperger's syndrome (AS) are milder during high school years, but your child might still benefit from services. It is hard to know what to ask for or understand what is reasonable for the school to provide. In the following sections, we give examples of some common accommodations, but please remember, the modifications he receives will be based on his unique needs. If you are having a hard time deciding what services or accommodations your child needs, consider requesting an updated evaluation.

Transitions from Grade to Grade

Transitions are more likely to pose challenges for an Aspie than they are for neurotypical children. Often more emphasis is placed on planning for and accommodating the small transitions that we see every day than for the big transitions that occur infrequently. Planning for transitioning to the next grade, to a new teacher, and even more importantly to the next school, is necessary. Having your child visit the new school prior to the start of the next school year is one important consideration to reduce his anxiety around the new environment. Even more important to his success is getting the new teaching staff to meet with the current teaching staff to share information that is not readily written down in the IEP documents. Although it doesn't always work, allowing new teachers to find out what has been tried and failed as well as what has been tried and succeeded can be incredibly beneficial for your child.

Elementary School

Many Aspies are successful during the elementary grades because social interactions are more straightforward, subjects in school are more concrete rather than abstract, and teachers in lower grades often have a more nurturing approach to teaching, accepting differences and teaching the same concept multiple ways to reach different learning styles. Even so, the following are examples of how schools can help young students.

During a normal school day, Aspies fight overwhelming sensory input, which can disrupt their ability to learn. Their need for order and structure also play an important role in how well they adjust in the classroom. The following are some minor adjustments teachers can make in the classroom environment:

- Allow more natural light or floor lamps in the classroom to limit exposure to fluorescent lighting.

- Allow modifications for sensory sensitivities, such as using glue sticks instead of paste.

- Provide a consistent daily schedule (in visual or picture form if applicable).

- Provide an area in the classroom where the student can go when feeling overwhelmed or near meltdown that is equipped with head-phones to block out noise and an enjoyable activity to reduce stress.

- Seat the child near the teacher or near supportive students who show strengths in areas the child has weaknesses.

- Provide designated areas that are clearly marked for books and belongings.

There are times throughout the school day when children move from class to lunch, or when in middle and high school, from class to class. These transitional times are hard for Aspies but can be made a little easier with a few changes:

- Provide extra time for transitions. For example, allow the student to leave for lunch or special classes a few minutes earlier than class-mates to minimize walking with crowds and to allow for extra time to organize materials when arriving at the special class.

- Institute a buddy system for transitional times of the day to help the child cope.

- Give the student advance notice of fire drills when possible or have earplugs to use during the extended drill.

- Provide advance notice of any changes of schedule.

Multisensory teaching methods such as demonstrations, hands-on activities, and using pictures as well as written text have been found to help increase learning in Aspies. In addition to making sure lessons include more than one sense, teachers can incorporate accommodations into their classrooms:

- Use social stories to teach social skills as well as practicing social skills in natural interactions, with the teacher observing and offering assistance.

- Allow extra time for completing written assignments and tests.

- Allow use of alternative methods of getting information into written format, like keyboarding or speech-to-text technologies.

- When communicating with the child, the teacher will use concrete and specific language, avoiding idioms, sarcasm, or vague terms such as "maybe" or "later."

- The teacher will use positive reinforcement programs, responding to attempts in a positive way.

- The teacher will create cooperative learning situations in which the child can share areas he is knowledgeable in.

Aides can help in a number of ways in the classroom, from monitoring behavior; to helping your child comprehend classroom rules; to making transitions; to helping with less supervised times such as in the hallway, lunch, or recess. Both the aide and teacher should be provided education on AS and allowed to consult with the special education teacher and/or the school district's autism specialist. Working with the school, you can help implement changes that help your child feel safe and secure and reach his potential.

MISC.

The Role of Aides

Your child's aide can be asked to be available to all students in a class during certain times of the day to take away some of the stigma of having a personal aide during class. Remember, the goal is normalization and having a one-on-one aide throughout the day is not normal. The aide should be reduced or eliminated as your child masters new skills and gains greater independence in completing tasks.

Middle School

Middle school proves difficult for many Aspies. More transitions occur during the day, and students are expected to take more responsibility for completing work. Teachers may not be familiar with how AS affects a student on a daily basis, assuming your child is immature, lazy, or unmotivated. Use the following suggestions as a starting point for creating a supportive and encouraging environment.

Some things for teachers to keep in mind when instructing Aspie children include:

- Provide social skills instruction.
- Provide visual cues when teaching how to summarize and write.
- Apply learning to real situations.
- Use concrete, specific language when discussing behavior.
- Incorporate the child's unique interests into teaching.

To address the difficulty Aspies have during transitions, teachers can allow students to …

- Leave the classroom a few minutes prior to or after other students to avoid problems in the hallway.
- Wear headphones to drown out loud noises or noisy hallways.

Suggestions to help Aspies keep up with the more demanding requirements of middle school include the following:

- Provide a checklist for weekly updates and waypoints.
- Utilize online calendars to post homework assignments and make assignments as specific as possible to avoid misinterpretation.
- Provide a weekly or monthly syllabus of what topics will be studied to help ease anxiety.

- Give copies of notes or allow students to copy from another student rather than taking notes during class. With the advent of Smart Boards and other technology, it is often very easy to provide the teacher's own notes in electronic format to your child using a flash drive.

- When having students work in groups, provide specific roles for each person in the group, with clear expectations and instructions.

The Doctor's Take Bullies are most prevalent during middle school years. You can include "protection from bullies" in your child's IEP and request an aide be nearby during lunch or recess time.

In addition to the suggestions listed here, care should be taken to make sure your child is not being disciplined for symptoms of AS. For example, Aspies are sometimes thought to be "talking back" or "being a smart aleck" when they answer based on literal thinking or because they refuse to make eye contact. Request informational sessions with teachers to explain how symptoms of AS show up in everyday social interactions, and make sure you have a system in place so you are aware immediately if your child's grades begin to slip.

Aspie Advice Some of the accommodations listed as suggestions for elementary schools may still be relevant during middle school and high school. Check through all of the accommodations and use those that are appropriate based on your child's needs rather than by age.

High School

During high school, the level of social interaction between teacher and student is limited, with students moving from class to class during the day. Teachers don't have as much opportunity to know each student on an individual basis, and because your child may be quiet, avoiding one-on-one interaction, teachers might view him as self-reliant or not having special needs. Make sure teachers are aware of your child's disability and ways they can reach out to help.

Aspies see the world in black and white. They need to make sense of what is said and have a hard time understanding abstract and complex concepts. Don't assume the student understood what has been said. Present information in short, simple sentences and paraphrase complex concepts in simpler language. Ensure understanding by having the student paraphrase or restate information and directions. Some ways for teachers to help Aspies when presenting lessons include:

- Pause between key points to give the student time to process the information.

- Ask only one question at a time.

- Prepare students ahead of time when having a substitute if possible.

- State clearly what is required.

- Break longer or complex tasks into manageable segments.

- Show examples whenever possible.

- Keep presentations written on the board as neat as possible.

When requesting accommodations, be as specific as possible. Explain exactly what you would like the teachers to do. Remember that regular and structured parent-teacher communication is just as important in high school as it is in the earlier grades. Set up a system of communication early in the year so you are immediately aware of any difficulties your child is having.

Sample IEP Goals

In addition to your child's IEP listing classroom accommodations, you and the IEP team will create specific goals that are considered necessary for your child's progress at school. These are unique to each child and are based on his evaluation or assessment, observations in the classroom, recommendations of teachers, and your input. Each goal is broken down into steps or objectives, and each one should be measureable as well as having a projected time the goal is expected to be met.

The Substitute Teacher Test

misc.

When developing IEP goals, ask yourself whether they pass the "substitute teacher test"—in other words, would someone without knowledge of your child be able to read the accommodations and goals and understand what to do? Because your child's IEP is relevant regardless of the teacher or who is implementing it, make sure words are unambiguous and directives are specific.

The following is an example of an IEP goal for a student with AS.

Will increase social communication skills by reaching benchmarks as outlined here:

1. Will initiate discussions, on topics other than their personal passion, with peers 3 out of 5 opportunities

2. Will compliment a peer 3 out of 5 opportunities

3. Will attempt to discover a peer's interests in 3 out of 5 discussions with peers

4. Will initiate varied topics of discussion during 3 out of 5 conversations with peers

5. Will take turns during a conversation with 3, and later 4, back-and-forth turns 3 out of 5 discussions with peers

6. Will ask questions of his conversation partner during 3 out of 5 discussions with peers

Each goal listed in the IEP should have specific objectives as this example does. At the annual review of your child's IEP, each goal should be reviewed for completion. Any goals not met should be reviewed for relevancy, and the team needs to decide whether further accommodations, services, or therapies need to be added to the IEP to help the student reach the goal.

Helping at Home

Although it is important to put into place classroom accommodations and goals within the IEP, it is also essential that you have strategies in place to help your child at home. The following sections provide tips and suggestions for parents.

Homework

Often an Aspie will want to write as little as possible, and this often leads to simply putting the answer down without showing his work. Help your child understand that showing his work has several advantages for him:

- It can result in more credit being given if his final answer is actually wrong.

- He has a chance of seeing where he made a mistake before the teacher discovers it.

- It helps develop skills that may be necessary later for harder work of the same type.

Provide your child a step-by-step example, showing exactly what information should be written on the paper.

Other ways to help include:

- Use visual organizers or timetables to help break large assignments or projects into smaller steps.

- Create a schedule for completing homework, having him do it at the same time each day and allowing a set amount of time for each topic. Help your child to focus on work scheduled for that time period. Incorporate small breaks into the homework schedule to avoid him being overwhelmed.

Aspie Advice

Sometimes Aspies have a hard time completing homework because it "doesn't make sense" to practice work he already understands. Talk about the importance of homework: it reinforces concepts and helps prepare him for times when he needs extra work on a topic. You can also explain that true mastery requires practice, and when he has mastered it completely, he will get the answers right and do them quickly. Accuracy and speed are the true signs of mastery.

- Some Aspies are afraid of making mistakes, to the degree that everything must be "perfect." They may spend an enormous amount of time erasing and rewriting to make sure there are no mistakes in their work. Sometimes simply telling them that hand-writing does not count as long as it is readable can cut down on this time-consuming process.

- Organize your child's work area. Clutter can annoy or distract him. Keep homework supplies, such as pens, pencils, rulers, and paper easily accessible.

Aspies who have rigid thinking may have a hard time completing home-work when it is not done or explained exactly like the teacher did it. For example, Tim was trying to finish his math homework. He didn't under-stand what to do, but when his mother tried to explain he became more frustrated, yelling that she was doing it wrong because his teacher did it differently. No matter how much his mother explained that the problem could be completed in more than one way, Tim was sure his homework would be wrong if it wasn't done exactly as his teacher had showed him.

Aspies may misunderstand directions or homework assignments. For younger children, talk to the teacher and request the names and phone numbers of two or three other students who can help him understand the assignment. The teacher may need to request permission from the parents before giving you phone numbers. You can also ask that homework assign-ments be emailed to you or be put up on an online calendar for review at night.

Study Skills

Many Aspies manage well academically and use exceptional abilities to help in areas that come less readily for them. For those who have a hard time with academics, the following tips can help:

- Understand how your child learns. Even though many Aspies are visual learners, not all are. Your child might learn best through hearing. Find out your child's learning style to help him develop strategies for studying.

- Use your child's passions to help explain concepts he doesn't understand.

> **MISC.**
>
> **Horses and Math**
>
> Carrie was passionate about all things horses, and she paid attention to schoolwork as long as her parents or teachers related it to horses. Math posed a particular challenge for her until horses were used as examples. Statistics were developed to analyze and predict crop yields, and therefore related to horses. Horse racing was used to explain distances and ellipses.

- As your child enters middle school and high school, help him plan his own homework times and break down projects rather than doing it for him.

Handwriting

Because Aspies may also have written expression disorder, which affects handwriting, it may be necessary to take extra time at home to help your child legibly write or hand in assignments the teacher can read.

- Whenever possible, have your child complete assignments on the computer.

- Use pencils and pens that are ergonomically designed—available from occupational therapy catalogues—to help relieve hand fatigue.

- Have your child do exercises before and after writing, such as rubbing hands together, shaking or flapping hands, stretching fingers apart then making a fist several times, to reduce tiredness from writing.

- See an occupational therapist to work with your child to help develop fine motor skills.

Monitoring Progress

When working with teachers and your child's IEP or educational team, discuss communication between home and school. It is important not only that you stay abreast of how your child is doing but that you are available to help solve problems that may occur at school.

> **The Doctor's Take**
>
> It was previously thought that bright Aspies were better off without homework. Experience has taught us differently. It is not possible to graduate with a genuine academic diploma without homework. College is no different. Homework should become a regular part of your child's life. Accommodations in *how* the work is done, such as typing, dictating, and breaking the project into smaller segments, are helpful, but minimizing or eliminating homework sends the wrong message. One of the most important lessons they can learn is that something does not have to be fun or come naturally to them to be important.

- First impressions are exceedingly important when working with people with Asperger's. Request a meeting with your child's new teachers during the preplanning days prior to students arriving at school for the first day. Help them get to know your child so they can make a positive impression on your child at their first meeting. This will significantly increase the chances of having a positive year.

- Request another meeting with your child's teachers within the first few weeks of school. Discuss your child's progress and what you hope to accomplish during the upcoming school year, both academically and socially. Let teachers know how they can help and that you are available should they have any questions.

- Set up a mode of communication at the beginning of the school year. You might prefer to have a weekly update by email or only receive notice if there is a problem. Be specific in what information you need to best help your child.

- Request a review of your child's educational services if you find he is having difficulty. If your child has an IEP or Section 504, it should be reviewed annually. However, you have a right to request a review at any time.

Keep communication open and positive with your child's teachers. Remember you are all part of a team working toward your child's success. View them as partners.

Essential Takeaways

- Your child's educational needs change as he grows and matures. Therefore, it is important to regularly review accommodations and services to make sure they are still relevant.

- Goals listed in your child's IEP should be clearly defined and list objectives or steps for reaching the goal.

- Parents can help at home by creating a homework schedule and having their child focus on one subject at a time.

- Create a mode of communication with teachers at the beginning of the school year to help monitor progress throughout the year.

chapter 18

Teaching Self-Help Skills

Finding ways to improve organization at school

Learning how to listen

Building conversations with scripts

Creating goals to monitor progress

From the time a child is born, parents try to instill skills to foster independence and self-reliance. When that child has a disability, such as Asperger's syndrome (AS), this is even more important. Skills learned in high school help prepare your child for adulthood, college, work, and future relationships. This chapter is meant to be shared with your preteen or teen Aspie, with strategies and suggestions to help him develop skills to use throughout his life.

Self-Help Skills at School

When your child is in elementary school, it is much easier to keep him organized and help him study for an upcoming test. As he moves into middle school, and then high school, it is normal if he resents you going through his backpack each night or pulling out papers to help keep him organized. He wants to be able to do these things on his own; it's just that symptoms of AS keep getting in his way.

Note Taking

Andrew never took notes. During class he listened intently to the teacher, and because he had a good memory, was able to pass his classes with high grades. When he did try to take notes, Andrew missed half of what his teacher said. He had a hard time figuring out what to write, so instead tried to write everything down in his notebook; while he was writing, the teacher continued his lesson, and after a few minutes, Andrew would get lost.

> **Aspie Advice**
>
> Explain to your teen that certain clues indicate information is important. For example, pay attention when the teacher writes something on the board, includes dates, gives specific procedures or directions, says facts more than once, tells the same information in more than one way, and gives an introduction or a summary of information. Notes should be taken in these situations.

Like many Aspies, Andrew had a problem figuring out what was important and what wasn't important. Because he had difficulty reading body language and inflections in voice, he missed the emphasis on certain facts and had no idea what to write down as important. As classes became more complex and notes were needed to study for tests, Andrew's grades started to slip. His parents knew note taking would be even more important in college and eventually in the workplace. At a minimum, he would some-day need to refer to important parts of conversations with his boss.

There are many different theories on the best way to take notes, but your teen needs to find the method that works best for him.

The following are several different strategies for taking notes; your teen might find one of these works well, or he may use a combination, creating his own system. It is important to try these methods out so he can choose the one right for him.

Ask the teacher if your child can record lectures. In the evening, he can listen to the recording again and take notes, stopping the recording to give him time to write. This strategy helps your teen learn how to take notes in a nonpressure environment. The first few times, you can listen to the recording with him and take your own notes; then compare to see whether he wrote down the important points.

The teacher can also supply notes, or even just the main points that will be discussed in class. Your teen follows along and adds notes to the basic outline, helping him understand what is important. Using this strategy, you can work with the teacher to, at first, supply full outlines of class notes and as the year progresses, put less in the outline, letting your child fill in larger amounts as he gets better at note-taking.

Draw a line down each notebook page, about one third of the way over from the margin. On the left side of the line, your teen writes down the main topic being discussed and on the right side of the line he writes supporting information.

Additional tips for your child to keep in mind when taking notes:

- Leave blank spaces on the paper so you can fill in additional information that you missed later.

- Write down phrases and keywords rather than full sentences.

- Skip writing examples unless you need the example to help you understand the concept.

- Reference pages in the text that can further illustrate a concept.

- Practice listening for voice inflections and gestures and write down information when your teacher's voice gets louder or he uses his hands to make a point.

- Experiment by sometimes using the teacher's words and sometimes using your own to see what is easier for you.

- If you miss something, don't worry about it. Leave a blank space on the page and continue taking notes. Ask your teacher (or another student) to help you fill in the blanks later.

Organization

While Aspies can be very organized, even overfocused on organization, in some areas (like their passion or hobby), they can also be very disorganized in other areas. Planning and organization are frequently difficult areas for Aspies. As one teen with AS said, "I never worry about the future; I only think about what is happening now." Looking to the future requires imagination, creating a vision of something that hasn't yet happened, which is hard for Aspies. To help him understand organization and planning, help your teen develop questions to ask himself when beginning a project or a class. The answers to these questions can help him develop an organizational structure. For example, in the beginning of the school year, have your teen answer the following questions for each class:

- What supplies do I need for this class?

- Do I need a binder or folder to hold loose papers?

- Do I need a separate notebook for each class, or is it better to use a binder with dividers so I am only carrying one item?

- If using a binder, would it be easier to have one binder for the entire day or two binders—one for morning classes and one for afternoon classes?

- Where do I put homework assignments to be handed in so I can always find them?

- What is the best way to keep track of assignments, test dates, and project due dates? Should I use an online calendar, an electronic organizer, or the calendar in my phone? Remember to consult with your child's school regarding which of these is acceptable. For example, many schools forbid the use of cellular phones during the academic day. You can have the use of a phone or electronic organizer placed in their IEP as an accommodation, if necessary.

- Would a second set of textbooks be a help? Often this can be written into the IEP as an accommodation for the student.

Use this strategy when planning activities or working on a school project. Creating questions in the present tense makes the situation seem relative in the moment rather than in the future and makes your teen think about what methods work best for him.

Using Technology

MISC.

Newer technologies can help greatly with organizational and paper management issues. A two-sided scanner is no longer something only high-tech offices can afford. Simple units that transform paper into Adobe PDF documents with Optical Character Recognition (OCR) technology are relatively cheap and can be used to create an exact copy for electronic storage, editing, or reproduction. Through the use of scanners, misplaced papers are less likely to be a problem, and ruining a page through overerasure or other mishaps is no longer a catastrophe because you can simply print out a second copy of the original.

Creating Lists

Every day we need to decide what is important and what tasks should be done and in what order. We frequently prioritize our daily tasks without giving it much conscious thought. We know what needs to be done and when it needs to be done. We can categorize our tasks as important to less important and can often do this without thinking much about it. Prioritizing, like planning, can be a weak skill for Aspies. One strategy, which can be used throughout your child's life, is to create daily to-do lists.

Have your teen use a notebook to write down tasks that must be completed, adding to the list throughout the day as he remembers something or as a new task comes up.

In the evening, have your teen write a "to-do" list for the following day, ranking each item in order of importance. He may want to incorporate other people's opinions of importance. For example, completing household chores might be way down on his idea of important; however, taking the trash out might be important because it is trash day.

As each item is completed, have your teen cross it out or put a check mark next to it. In the evening, move any tasks that have not been completed to the next day's to-do list.

Additional tips:

- Have your teen get in the habit of reviewing his list each morning, at lunch, and again in the evening to check on his progress and to complete any tasks he forgot about.

- For some tasks, there might be deadlines. Include this information on the list so he can see at a glance how much time is left to complete the task.

Remind your teen that lists are an important part of keeping track of tasks, but that the list must also be flexible, leaving time for new tasks that come up as well as priorities changing. Give him real-life examples of how your priorities often change through the day and week at work and at home.

Social Skills

We have talked about social skills throughout this book, but in this section we discuss some exercises and specific ways for teaching your teen how to improve listening and conversation skills.

Effective Listening

Effective listening, like many other social skills, can be learned and shows others that they are important to you. Listening skills use your entire body to convey that you are interested. Your teen can take a number of steps to show he is listening. There are also ways to interpret the speaker's feelings.

The Doctor's Take

Help your child understand that listening to others talk about themselves has several distinct advantages for him: people view those who listen rather than talk as more likeable, listening helps you learn about others and know who to go to when you need help, listening helps you develop new ways of telling stories or saying things, and you might learn about a new topic of interest.

Pay attention to what his body language says:

- Try to incorporate subtle movements, such as leaning his body toward the speaker, facing the other person squarely, keeping arms and legs uncrossed, and nodding his head during the conversation.

- Maintain the proper distance, approximately 3 feet or one arm's length. Too much distance makes it seem you want to get away; too little distance can be intimidating.

Pay attention to the speaker's body language:

- What does their facial expression say? Is the speaker smiling, conveying enjoyment? Is he frowning, showing unhappiness about the topic?

- How does the speaker's tone of voice match what they are saying? Is his voice high pitched, showing excitement or anger? Is he speaking with different voice inflections, showing interest?

- How is the speaker holding his body? Is he stiff, showing dissatisfaction or irritation? Is his body relaxed, showing his enjoyment or interest in the conversation?

Teach your child to use reflective listening—restating what the person has said in his own words. When he repeats what the person says, he not only validates that he has listened, he verifies that he heard correctly. He can restate by saying something like "If I have heard you correctly, you feel …" or "Do I understand you? You feel …"

Role-Playing and Using Scripts

Role-playing is when two or more people "act out" a social situation to practice skills in a risk-free setting. Role-playing is usually based on a hypothetical scenario but one that is similar to real-life situations. This gives your teen the ability to "be" different people within the scene so he gains perspective on how the different people involved in the social situation feel.

Aspie Advice
Many times parents don't understand what is currently important to teens. This makes listening to other teens important. The last thing you want is for your Aspie teen to sound *more* like an adult! So a slightly older teen who is both socially skilled and helpful is a very important resource. They are going to help you develop scripts that improve your child's chances of naturally slipping into conversations with peers.

Gary had trouble initiating conversations. He was okay when others came up to him and started talking, but if no one did, he would sit by himself rather than having to start a conversation. He had no idea what to say, and if he tried, the words never seemed to come out right. It was easier to not try. Gary's parents worked with him on creating a number of "conversation starters"—such as those discussed in Chapter 10—both general ones and some topics he knew were of interest to his classmates, such as baseball.

Gary and his parents took turns being a classmate so that Gary had a chance to practice the phrases he had made up, such as "Hi, Matt, did you see that baseball game on television last night?" He practiced different ways of saying hello and different questions to ask until he felt a little more comfortable. Gary also took a turn playing his classmates while his father pretended to be Gary, to give him some perspective of how the classmate would feel when someone came up and talked to him. Gary began to understand that just as he appreciated someone starting the conversation, his classmates might feel the same way.

After role-playing several times, Gary wrote up a longer script, filling in what he thought his classmates might say and how he could respond. He knew the conversation would probably not go exactly the same, but it gave him some ideas. He especially focused on coming up with questions about different topics he had heard classmates talk about. Besides baseball, he had heard them discussing other sports, music, and their school classes.

The next day, Gary tried out one of his scripts. He was really scared but decided to start with Matt, who had the locker next to him and liked baseball. There was a game on the previous night, and this morning Gary had made sure to check the score on the news before heading off to school. "Hey, Matt, did you see the baseball game last night on television?" Gary said, just like he had practiced.

"No, but I heard our team won by three points. It was on pretty late; I had to go to bed," Matt replied.

"Me, too, but I saw some of the highlights on the news this morning. It looked like a good game." Gary felt a little more confident, and the conversation continued for a few more minutes before they had to go into class.

When meeting new people or talking to classmates, scripts are a great way for your teen to have a ready resource of topics to talk about. You may want to work on several different scripts, for example, asking for help, talking to someone you don't know, or disclosing the diagnosis of AS. As your teen continues to practice and use scripts, his speech will sound more natural, and although it may not be completely comfortable for him, he should feel more confident at starting a conversation.

Self-Assessment

One of the most important aspects of self-help skills is to be able to monitor progress and make corrections when necessary. Your teen can begin to monitor his new skills in a number of different ways. Academic skills are obviously easier to monitor because you receive grades and feedback from teachers on a regular basis. If poor note-taking skills had resulted in poor test grades and after working on taking better notes test scores improved, then strategies worked. But monitoring progress in social skills is not as easy because there is often no concrete measurement.

Setting Goals

In the example of Gary creating scripts, he and his parents set a goal of Gary initiating at least one conversation with a classmate each week to give Gary something specific to work toward. Setting goals such as this is a good way to measure progress. Goals, however, need to be set correctly in order to work. The following are steps you can share with your teen for setting effective goals:

1. Choose one goal at a time—choosing more makes it confusing and overwhelming.

2. Make your goal specific and measurable. A statement such as "I will make more friends" is not a goal; it is a vague statement that can have different interpretations. The goal Gary and his parents made, "I will initiate one conversation per week on a topic other than my personal favorite" is both specific—it tells Gary exactly what he needs to do—and measurable because it gives both a number and time limit. At the end of the week, Gary will know if he met the goal.

3. Write down the goal. This helps to further your commitment to the goal.

4. Create a plan of action. Write down the steps you need to take to reach the goal. In Gary's goal, he needed to create scripts and role-play before going to school and trying to initiate the conversation. Knowing each step helps keep you focused.

5. Reward progress. Think of something your teen wants to do and use this as a reward for reaching a goal. It could be buying something related to his interest or could be extra computer time. Having something to look forward to helps keep him motivated.

> **The Doctor's Take**
>
> When setting goals, make sure expectations are reasonable and goals are achievable. When goals are unrealistic, they foster a sense of failure rather than one of success.

Remember, as with anything in life, there are bound to be setbacks and disappointments. Don't be too hard on your teen. Review the goal to make sure it is realistic. If it is, find out whether the setback is something external, or if there is an additional step that would benefit your teen.

Video Assessments

When working with scripts and role-playing, it is helpful to videotape the sessions. You and your teen can look over the video and see what he did right and what he could change. Although it isn't advisable to have him videotape classmates, you may be able to record your child interacting with people at church, at clubs, or with neighbors to let him observe his own body language and that of the other person. He can compare how he looked and acted when you first started practicing scripts and how he looks after several weeks or months of practicing conversations.

Another way of self-monitoring is creating checklists of what needs to be done during a conversation and having your teen check off items that he completed and continue practicing those areas he did not do well.

Here are some potential checklist items:

❑ Make eye contact with your partner.

❑ Stay on topic.

❑ Use appropriate voice volume.

❑ Use appropriate nonverbal communication.

❑ Ask questions about the other person.

❑ Make comments.

❑ Take turns.

❑ Demonstrate appropriate personal space.

❑ Be respectful.

❑ Begin and end conversation appropriately.

MISC.

Ending Conversations

It is important to help your child end a conversation. First, he may tend to dominate a conversation, and recognizing this and ending the conversation can get him a second chance with that person. Second, he will get into conversations that make him uncomfortable. Third, he may realize that he is going to be late if he continues to listen without leaving. Use the skills already discussed to develop scripts for your child to use if he needs to end a conversation.

Self-assessment is used by adults in many areas of life. At work, they assess their strengths and weaknesses and search out ways to improve those areas they need help in, such as adult learning classes or by reading books. Teaching your teen to use various self-assessment tools will benefit him throughout his life.

Essential Takeaways

- Aspies may have trouble taking notes because they have a hard time distinguishing what is important from what is not.

- Effective listening involves paying attention to what is said and what is not said and showing the speaker you are interested in what he is saying.

- Role-playing is acting out a hypothetical situation to allow practice of social skills in a risk-free environment.

- Self-assessment skills, such as setting and monitoring goals, will help your teen throughout his life.

chapter 19

Considerations for College

Exploring college opportunities

Preparing for accommodations

Additional ways parents can help

Preparation for college should begin when your teen is still in high school. For those children with IEPs, transitional plans are included in the goals; your child may have had training on social skills, organizational skills, and daily life skills to help him in getting ready to live on his own. Students with Asperger's syndrome (AS) frequently struggle with balancing independence with continued reliance on their parents. Some may want to go off to college to prove they can manage on their own.

Heading off to College or Vocational School

For students with IEPs, many states offer vocational assessment services to students over 16 to help them make more informed decisions about possible school and work options after high school. It is very important that you check with your child's high school for what services and evaluations are available to help your child plan and transition to life after high school. You should contact the school well before it's time to make such decisions, often as much as two to three years before graduation.

Choosing a School

Many things must be considered when choosing the right school for your child. While many people think of college as an "all or nothing" move, living at a traditional four-year college is not the only option. Some of your other choices are:

Community college. These colleges offer two-year Associate degree programs in a variety of subjects, and many also have numerous certificate programs available. These offer a chance to experience college while still living at home and receiving support.

Specialty schools. A specialty school usually offers certificate programs in a narrow area, such as culinary arts, cosmetology, or graphic arts. Some have dormitories; others are strictly for commuters.

Technical or vocational schools. These schools offer training in a shorter time than college programs and offer choices for training in computer repair or programming, heating and air conditioning, or other trades.

Online courses. Some colleges specialize in online education, giving your teen a chance to continue his education from home.

Aspie Advice
Before sending your teen off to college, have him complete a learning style assessment. Knowing how he learns—visually, auditory, kinesthetic—can help him create study strategies. There are also often options to visit the school, sometimes for a summer camp or other activity, that will allow him to live in a dorm on campus for a few days.

If your child does decide to attend a four-year college, he still has choices. He can take classes part-time while working part-time; commute to a local college and receive support at home, or attend and live at college. Many colleges are now more understanding of students with special needs and are willing to make accommodations for students with AS.

When visiting colleges, call ahead to make an appointment with the disability services office to find out how they can help. General information you receive about accommodations or modifications might be specifically for those with physical disabilities; ask what types of supports are available specifically for students with AS. Use this time to find out whether there are support groups or social skills training. Some colleges have peer mentoring programs to help students get oriented to college life.

Colleges and universities usually offer a broad range of majors, but may focus in one or two specific areas. Look for schools that offer extended course work that matches your child's passion. Knowing that course work will include information about his passion can help motivate him not only when looking for schools but during the first few stressful months.

Planning for Daily Living

During the college years, your child not only needs to work on specific studies, he needs to learn how to take care of himself and behave as an adult. It will be necessary for him to possess time-management skills and complete daily living tasks. Before your child heads off to live in the dorm, make sure he knows how to do his own laundry and shop for personal hygiene products. Even if he has opted to stay at home and go to college, at this age you should be encouraging self-care behaviors.

> **The Doctor's Take**
>
> Create a list of important information for your child: phone numbers of the disability services office, his academic advisor, a list of his professors including their office locations and phone numbers, and where the counseling office is located. Also provide a copy of his schedule, a campus map marked to show buildings he will be going to on a regular basis, and any other important information or documents. Place everything in a folder that he can keep in his room or backpack for reference.

Another area in which your child may need help is time management. He needs to know when and where to study and how to schedule time each day for reviewing information and completing any assignments. He needs to keep track of test dates, assignments, and project due dates. Making sure your child has a large calendar to hang on his wall might help him track what he needs to do. After he has his class schedule, you, or a peer mentor, can work with him on creating a daily schedule.

Requesting Services and Accommodations

During the high school years, it is the school's responsibility to identify students with special needs and develop accommodations and modifications to help. Although colleges offer accommodations for students, it is up to the student to request any additional services. This is done through the disability services office and requires documentation of a disability, and the college may request additional documentation on suggested accommodations or information on why certain accommodations are needed.

> MISC.
>
> **Requesting Accommodations**
>
> Many parents think that having services and accommodations in high school automatically qualifies their child for services in college, but this is not true. Sometimes the eligibility material from the public school will be sufficient, occasionally a physician's letter is required, but a current evaluation is usually necessary. In some states, public colleges offer assessments. Check with the disability office in the college to find out what additional information is needed.

Some Aspies prefer not to ask for accommodations, instead trying to "make it on their own." If they find they need accommodations later, it is still possible to request them. However, professors are only required to offer the accommodations from that date forward; any changes or modifications are not retroactive.

Accommodations are specific to your child's needs, and there are no set accommodations a student will receive. Some request ideas are:

- Having a single room instead of sharing a room with a roommate
- Having a peer mentor
- Developing a crisis plan
- Offering tutoring or writing lab services
- Allowing extended time for tests
- Having additional access to professors
- Options to type tests instead of using pen/pencil

Talk with your child about what accommodations he feels are appropriate and will be helpful to him. Use the previous suggestions as well as reviewing any accommodations he had in high school to create a list he can discuss with the disabilities office. Some accommodations do not need to go through the disabilities office, but instead are plans you and your child put into place to make living at college easier.

It might sound like common sense, but before you drop your child off at the dorm and head back home, take some time to make sure he is oriented with the campus. Make sure he has a map of the campus and has marked where his classes are located. You might want to take the time to mimic his days, walking through the campus as he would to get from class to class. It will likely go a long way to making you both feel more comfortable.

Ongoing Parental Support

Whether your teen is going to be living on campus or staying home, he will need your continued support. The first year of college is stressful for all students, and he may find it hard to cope with the many different pressures; at the same time he may resent you being involved and reject any of your advice. Keep in touch with him by email and phone without inundating him and respect his right to find his own way. If he asks for help, try to offer suggestions but allow him to make the choice on what he thinks is best.

Sometimes, as parents, you need to allow him to "sink or swim," making him take responsibility for his actions and encouraging him to deal with what happens if he doesn't complete his work or spends too much time working on one assignment over another. It is very important to know as a parent that after your child is off at college you may have limited access to information about him while he is away. You may not be able to access his grades, even if you are financially responsible.

Some parents find using a life coach helps. A coach works on helping your child manage his weaknesses and focus on his strengths while giving encouragement. Instead of telling your child what to do, a coach listens and helps him talk through his choices. Coaches can also help work on specific problems, such as organization or communication skills.

Coaches work via email or telephone and usually have set appointments on a weekly basis, but many are also available for emergency situations in between normal sessions.

Talk to your child about the changes in your relationship and what parts of his life you will continue to be actively involved in. Explain that he will need to take care of daily living tasks on his own, making sure he eats regularly, taking his own medication, doing his laundry, and waking up in time for class. He may still want you to help him to choose classes each semester; be sure to give advice but resist the urge to make all the decisions for him. Instead ask questions and offer suggestions and then let him make the final decision.

> **The Doctor's Take**
>
> Most colleges offer supports and services through the health center and/or the counseling center. Often there are classes on time management, social skills, career planning, and how to navigate the curriculum. If your child has been receiving therapy for issues related to his AS, he may be able to receive the same type of therapy through the counseling center for little or no cost. An additional benefit of connecting with the counseling center is that they can be more responsive to your child in the event of a crisis.

On other matters, such as health care, you may still want to be involved. Because your child is now considered legally an adult, doctors and other medical professionals are bound by privacy laws and cannot share information with you. Preparing a health care proxy and having your child sign it gives medical providers the right to talk to you about health care issues. If your child has ongoing health concerns, this may be a good idea.

It is important to know that the restrictions on mental health information are significantly greater than on traditional medical and surgical information. Make certain that if you need to be involved in any mental health–related services, whatever release or authorization you have meets that state's requirements to access mental health information, not merely "all medical and surgical" information.

Set up a specific time to check in with your child. When he heads off to college, you feel a loss. You have invested an enormous amount of time and energy into your child's well-being; most days you were wrapped up in making sure his needs were met and worrying about his future. Now the house seems quiet, and you aren't sure what to do with your time. You want to check in every day to make sure he is okay. But this probably isn't what is best for him. He needs to stand on his own and can't do that if you are calling constantly and helping him decide what to do. Instead, choose a time once or twice a week to call and talk. Let him know he can call (or text) in between if something comes up.

If you have requested a private dorm room for your child, he will have a place to go to be alone, to unwind, or to hide during times of extreme stress or when he feels a meltdown coming on. If your child is living with someone else, he won't always have this "alone space" to work through high emotional times. Talk with him about what he can do and where he can go. You might suggest talking with the dormitory advisor about quiet places in the dorm he can go to when he needs to be alone, or the counseling office might offer some suggestions. Often students can reserve a study carrel or booth in the library, but these may require a reservation or prior arrangements. Being prepared for these moments helps make him feel more in control in a new and scary world.

Just as preparation and role-playing were important in high school, they still can help as your child ventures out into the world. Help your child look at clubs, organizations, and activities available at his college and suggest he attend different meetings before deciding on a few to join. Review and role-play ways to start a conversation and how to introduce himself to new people. Go over how to ask for help and how to respond when someone asks him for assistance.

Be sure you let your child know that your home is always his home. If going away to college was a bad decision, you can revise the plan and have him return home. But be sure you aren't setting up your child for failure, accepting that he can decide to come home as soon as college life becomes difficult. You need to balance your unconditional support with a belief that he is capable of succeeding at college.

Essential Takeaways

- Review the different types of schools and opportunities that are available to help your child make the best decisions.

- By college age, your child should be encouraged to participate in self-care behaviors, such as doing laundry or shopping for personal hygiene products.

- Contact the disability services office to discuss documentation needed to receive accommodations at college.

- Your child will need your continued support even when away at college, but you must also allow him to accept the consequences of his actions.

You and Your Family

Even though your child has Asperger's syndrome (AS), it affects your entire family. In Part 6 we talk about family relationships and how to maintain your relationship while raising a child with special needs. We help you and your spouse understand the process of acceptance, starting with denial and letting go of guilt.

Children with AS need structure, but how much is too much? We discuss the need for balancing structure with flexibility and setting rules that are "Asperger-friendly." One effective discipline method is using a token economy, and we provide a step-by-step guide to creating a token economy in your house.

Attending events with your Aspie is always an adventure, but we give you suggestions to help lessen the stress and make the day—or days—go more smoothly. We also offer guidelines for talking to friends and relatives about your child's diagnosis.

chapter 20

Taking Care of You and Your Marriage

When a parent can't accept the AS diagnosis

Finding time for yourself

Reducing stress

Keeping your marriage together

For each of us, a number of moments are forever burned into our minds—moments we can recall in detail, the time, the place, and how we felt. Being told your child has Asperger's syndrome (AS) might be one of those times. How did you feel? Were you devastated, or were you relieved? In this chapter, we talk about getting past the diagnosis, keeping some sense of normalcy in your family life, and making sure your marriage survives.

The Process of Acceptance

Dina walked out of the doctor's office in shock. Asperger's syndrome? Autism? Those were the words her son's pediatrician threw around. What did this mean? Was her son, Sammy, destined to be disabled his whole life? Even though the doctor had taken extra time to explain the diagnosis, Dina was left with many unanswered questions. She had heard of autism and AS, of course, and a few women in her circle of acquaintances had children with one or the other, but that was the extent of her knowledge. The pediatrician had recommended a full evaluation by a specialist to determine whether her son did have AS.

Denial

Dina's first thought was that the doctor must be wrong. She began to think about her son's behaviors and looked at all the things he could do. He could talk, even had an advanced vocabulary, sometimes sounding like a miniature adult. He focused on and cared about his schoolwork, taking time each night to make sure it was done correctly. He still had tantrums; sometimes they were pretty bad, but the tantrums normally happened when he was frustrated because he couldn't do something—that was normal, wasn't it?

> **Aspie Advice**
>
> You may feel a sense of loss when given a diagnosis of AS for your child. From the moment he was born, you envisioned his life, and now you feel all of your dreams and plans have been dashed. Remember, many people with AS lead successful, happy lives. Keep a positive attitude and allow your child to create his own life. Although this is a normal reaction, if you continue to feel grief or sadness for an extended time, talk with your doctor.

Dina's husband had the same reaction—"No way, he's just really smart and doesn't have many friends because he is smarter and more mature than the other kids his age. Don't worry, he'll be fine." And to her husband, that was the end of it. But the doctor's words kept swirling around Dina's mind; she decided before she made up her mind she would do some research. She talked to the women she knew who had children with AS, and the behaviors they described sounded pretty similar to Sammy's behaviors. She went online and read website after website on AS. Although there was a lot of confusing and often contradictory information online about AS, to her surprise the more she read, the more she believed AS might be a possibility. Her next step was to make an appointment with the specialist and to convince her husband the evaluation was a good idea.

AS is a life-changing diagnosis and the "not my child" reaction is natural; it is difficult to admit there is "something wrong" with your child. Many parents might have spent years making excuses such as "he's tired" or have learned to work around the symptoms. Some may blame one another for their child's behavior, accusing their partner of being too strict or too lenient. While you are exploring the possibility of an AS diagnosis, it is important to try to come to an agreement with your spouse. Working together is in the best interest of your child.

So what do you do if your partner doesn't even want to consider AS? Instead of trying to talk to him about the diagnosis, shift the conversation to the evaluation. Agree that your child may not have AS, and the doctor may be overreacting. Focus on having your partner agree only to scheduling an assessment and leave the conversation on the diagnosis until after you receive the results of the evaluation and know what diagnosis you are dealing with. Point out that there is a possibility the evaluation will prove him correct, and the whole thing will go away. Ask your spouse to agree to talk with the specialist after the evaluation is complete. Later in this chapter, we talk more about when you and your partner don't agree on how to manage AS.

What About the Guilt?

When a diagnosis is official, the next natural question is, "Did I do this?" You begin to look back, examine the pregnancy—what you ate, what you did. You look at your child's early years. Did you push him too hard? Did you yell too often? Did you not do enough for him? Did you do too much? Although no one knows the exact cause of AS, we do know that poor parenting does not cause it. There is evidence that it is, at least in part, hereditary. Studies have shown that siblings of children with autism or AS have a higher chance of having it as well, and some parents have discovered they have AS after learning about the symptoms through their child's diagnostic process.

MISC.

Why Is Diagnosis Important?

An "official" diagnosis does not change who your child is or how you feel about him. But a diagnosis is not just a label, either. An evaluation should result in a diagnosis and tailored recommendations (supports, treatments, and other resources) to make your child's life, and yours, easier. There is a wide array of supports and interventions that can help, but coming to grips with the need for them is part of starting down a positive road of change.

Trying to figure out the cause of AS isn't the only reason parents feel guilty. Some of the other reasons include ...

You handled situations wrong before the diagnosis. This is especially true when your child isn't diagnosed until preteen or teen years. You think back on all the times you lost your patience and yelled at him for meltdowns or for not listening. You feel guilty that you punished him for "being an Aspie."

You worry that your other children aren't receiving enough attention because so much time and effort go into taking care of your Aspie. Now that you have an official diagnosis, you will add doctor's visits, therapist visits, and meetings with the school. You feel guilty that you depend on your other children to take on more responsibility.

You compare yourself to other parents with Aspies, and somehow you never live up to what they are doing. The woman down the street spends more time working with her son; she volunteers more at school; she takes a walk with him every evening. Another acquaintance has a son with AS who is on the honor roll and tells you the secret is to make sure you let him do as much as he can by himself—don't hover over him. You don't know whether you are doing too much or too little. Remember, each child with AS is unique and has individual needs that may not be the same as the boy down the street. Focus on your own child's needs and what works for him, instead of comparing your strategies with another parent's.

How could you not have known there was something wrong? After all, you are the parent; you are supposed to know these things, supposed to be aware of all your child's needs. You feel that you have let him down, especially if he is diagnosed as a preteen or teen. You have heard that Early Intervention (EI) is the key to success, and because you weren't observant enough, your child didn't have any therapies in early childhood. Don't worry; many children with AS don't get EI services because children with AS aren't usually diagnosed before the age of 3. In the United States, the average age for diagnosis is between 11 and 12 years old.

Guilt can cripple you and stop you from giving your family what they need. It can drive you to spend every moment learning about AS and ignoring the actual needs of your family. Guilt can fill you with worry and paralyze you from taking action or push you into mindless frenetic action. Take time to understand the diagnosis and the strategies that are outlined in this book. Then move on to the next step, acceptance, and actively work to help your child and your family.

Acceptance

Welcome to your new "normal." An AS diagnosis will probably change your family's daily life, but you have already been dealing with the symptoms of AS and have already figured out many ways to help your child. A diagnosis of AS doesn't change how you feel about your child; you loved him before, and you love him now. A diagnosis gives you the opportunity to better understand how your child thinks and how to react to frustrating behaviors. It gives you a chance to create a plan of action and move forward.

It's Just Asperger's!

misc.

Many parents and Aspies are relieved when they are given a diagnosis of AS. Finally, they understand the rigid thinking, the quirky behaviors. Finally, parents understand why their children don't seem to listen, and children understand that they aren't crazy—they just have AS.

Acceptance means you are ready to admit weaknesses are associated with a diagnosis of AS, find solutions, and work to help your child be the best he can be. It means you are open to learning how to best help your child and seeking out resources, organizations, and professionals to help you better understand and work with your child's strengths. When you accept your child with AS, you embrace his differences. Review your expectations, making sure they are realistic but allow for your child's continued growth. But most of all, acceptance means that you continue to love and cherish your child.

Making Time for Yourself

Raising a child with special needs is time consuming and can be mentally and emotionally exhausting. Your days are filled with medical appointments, meetings with teachers, monitoring homework, and managing symptoms of AS. If your child is involved in activities, you probably spend time getting him there and back home. And if you have other children, daily responsibilities are doubled or tripled. Besides the time you spend taking care of your child, you still need go to work every day and/or take care of all the household responsibilities. Finding time for yourself and your marriage is probably way down on your priorities, but it is imperative that you create ways to relieve stress, focus on your needs, and keep your marriage healthy and strong.

Although your Aspie may need extra attention and more of your time than your other children, you need to devote time to your interests and find ways to keep up with friendships. This time helps you recharge— mentally, physically, spiritually, and emotionally—allowing you to give more to your family when you are with them. Without giving yourself space, you may end up resenting your child because AS has taken so much away from you; as you let friendships slip away, you may feel alone. Taking time for yourself sends a message to your family: your needs are important. By respecting yourself, you show family members you expect their respect as well.

Managing Stress

Even before your child was diagnosed with AS, life at your house was probably exhausting. Meltdowns, constant questions, fights with siblings or classmates have left you feeling drained. While other parents were able to take a few minutes for themselves while their child was occupied or felt confident leaving a child with a relative or babysitter, you didn't. Your child doesn't take well to other people, and babysitters are never sure how to handle the odd behaviors. Without an outlet, stress has made you irritable, angry, or easily frustrated but can also have produced physical symptoms, such as headaches, body aches, tiredness, and problems sleeping. The following ideas can help relieve stress.

Aspie Advice

It is not unusual for parents to sacrifice their own physical and emotional needs for their child. But your child needs you to be at your best, both physically and emotionally. Taking care of yourself is a gift you give your child.

Keep track of what increases your stress levels. Pay attention to the physical signs of stress so you can take steps to help you relax before feeling overwhelmed. For example, if meltdowns are hard for you to handle, and you notice your neck muscles tensing as your child's frustration level goes up, plan for this stress. Besides creating steps to help your child manage feeling overwhelmed, write down steps you can take, such as deep breathing, reminding yourself your child's meltdown is a way of communicating with you, and focusing on a solution rather than the meltdown itself.

Look for a support group, either locally or online. Nothing is more helpful than being able to talk about what is going on in your family to people you know will understand. It is hard to unleash your frustrations with friends and relatives who don't have any concept of living with an Aspie, but parenting support groups give you a sense that you are not alone and that others understand exactly what you are going through.

Accept that you can't be everything to everybody. We are often caught up in the "super parent" cycle, faulting ourselves if we can't meet every family member's need immediately. Understand that a family works together to meet needs, and it is not your role to jump to solve any and all problems that arise. Help teach family members independence and encourage them to take responsibility for their own needs as much as possible.

Exercise and consistent restful sleep are the two best stress fighters. The research is clear—regular moderate exercise and consistent restful sleep can do more to combat the effects of stress than medications, therapy, and other artificial supports. Although additional supports may be necessary from time to time, remember that regular exercise and consistent restful sleep are not optional extras in your life.

Schedule "me" time into every day. Hide in your bedroom for 15 minutes and let everyone know you are unavailable unless an emergency occurs (remember to define emergency). Take a bath, read a book, work in the garden; do whatever it is that helps you relax and demand your family respect this short break.

Make a list of supportive people in your life. You need to be able to reach out to others during times of high stress, but you don't want to reach out to those who judge you or your child. Having a list handy helps you call the right people. For example, you might call your sister every day, but when you talk about problems with your son, you end up feeling worse; your cousin, however, just listens and lets you know she is there for you. Make sure you have phone numbers of those who are supportive handy and call them when feeling overwhelmed.

> **The Doctor's Take**
>
> It is common for parents of an Aspie to develop stress. You may get irritable, display low mood, and have difficulty focusing. Don't dismiss that you can benefit from the support of a professional in dealing with stress. Remember, all therapists aren't created equal. You want someone who is competent and someone with whom you are comfortable discussing embarrassing issues. Counseling should help you deal with current issues and give you new skills to help you better manage your stress going forward.

Spend alone time with each child every day. You don't need to have an extended time together to let each of your children know you love them. Ensuring you spend 10 minutes reading a story, playing a game, or talking, and giving each one your undivided attention during that time helps all your children know you love them unconditionally.

Give a compliment. Get into the habit of looking for reasons to compliment someone. This can be the bank teller, the cashier at the grocery store, and members of your own family. Giving a compliment boosts both your mood and the receiver's mood. This has the additional benefit of showing your Aspie how to give and receive compliments, an area that is sometimes difficult to master.

Make arrangements to do something outside of the house for yourself. Go for a manicure or a massage, meet friends for lunch, join a gym, take a class, or go for a walk after dinner each night. Removing yourself from the situation helps you keep a more positive perspective.

Incorporate stress-reducing activities into your family time. Chances are you are not the only one in the family feeling stress, your partner and your children feel the pressure of living in an Aspie household. Set aside quiet reading time, take a family walk, play a board game together, have family exercise time, or make cleaning the house a family game—put on music and give each person responsibilities and sing and dance while cleaning. Make sure you choose activities that will be fun and relaxing; don't try to make stressful activities fun.

Make sure you enlist the help of your partner, explaining that sometimes you need some personal time and would like him to hold down the fort during those times, but that you are willing to do the same for him.

Laugh

MISC.

There is nothing as relaxing as laughing. Enjoy the moment; find the humor in the situation. The logical, linear thinking of children with AS often provides funny interactions—rather than being frustrated with his inability to understand, enjoy his unique sense of viewing the world.

Maintaining Your Relationship with Your Spouse

As the responsibilities in your family increase, the time for you and your spouse to have fun together decreases. Before your children were born, each evening was spent sharing the highlights of your day and focusing on one another's needs, but now both of you spend your evenings making dinner, helping with homework, being taxi driver, and dealing with behavioral issues, leaving little energy for your relationship. But the added stress of having a child with special needs makes a strong relationship even more important. You need to be able to talk about school problems and behavioral issues and find strategies that both of you feel comfortable with.

You and your spouse might accept that whatever time is left after all your family responsibilities are completed belong to you as a couple, but too often once everything is done, one or both of you are ready to collapse into bed, grabbing a few hours of sleep before the chaos starts over again the next day. By doing so, you and your spouse are showing your family and one another that your relationship isn't important and doesn't deserve attention. Instead, make it clear that no matter how important children, jobs, and activities are, your relationship is most important by making time for each other every day.

Make a decision to spend time being together. You might turn off the television and talk to each other after the children are in bed or wake up half an hour before the children get up to enjoy a peaceful cup of coffee together. Make sure your "together time" isn't filled with discussions about children, school, or discipline. Instead, talk about dreams, plans for the future, and interests you share; make this a special time during which you connect with one another.

If you and your spouse are feeling overwhelmed with a new diagnosis of AS, meltdowns, or school issues, you might find it hard to be positive or feel loving toward one another. Think back to your early relationship and remember why you married your spouse. What attracted you to him? What traits did you see as special? If you need to, write a list of why you love your spouse and read it over when you are feeling unconnected. You might want to give him a copy of your list and ask him to write one listing the reasons he loves you. It helps to focus on the reasons you are together instead of focusing on your different viewpoints.

Find ways to go on a date with your spouse. If you don't have close friends or relatives you feel safe leaving your child with, be creative. Set up a fancy dinner in your living room after the children are in bed or take a day off work and spend it together when the children are in school. If you can find a babysitter, make a pact to go on a date at least one night per month (once a week is better but may not be doable). Use this time to explore shared interests or create new ones; for example, take a ballroom dancing class together. Romance may not be as spur of the moment as it was in the beginning of your relationship, but that doesn't make it any less loving. Your marriage is worth the effort.

Agree to Disagree

MISC.

If you and your spouse don't agree on discipline for your child, agree to disagree—in private. Resist the urge to correct your partner in front of your children and ask for the same respect from your spouse. You can discuss your differences later and work toward a compromise.

If you and your spouse don't agree on how to raise your Aspie, one of you may be in denial, or you just don't agree on discipline methods. Your child will be better off if you and your spouse are on the same page, but this often takes a lot of effort and compromise. We talk more about specific discipline methods in Chapter 21, but the following tips can help you and your spouse work together:

- Find a local support group and go to meetings together, learning how other parents handle certain situations and then discussing alternatives to find common ground.

- Talk about the positive traits of AS and accept your child's quirky or odd characteristics as part of his personality.

- Learn about AS together so you better understand why your child behaves in a certain way or says certain things to help prevent anger before it begins.

- Reword thoughts about your child. Instead of saying, "Why won't he listen to me?" use the words, "What is he trying to communicate?" By rephrasing this, you and your spouse can move from anger over a situation to problem-solving.

If, no matter what you try, your marriage continues to deteriorate and both of you are unhappy, you might want to consider talking with a marriage counselor, minister, or marriage coach. Sometimes talking with a neutral party can help both of you find common ground and learn to work together with this new and challenging situation.

Essential Takeaways

- Denial is a common reaction when parents are first given a diagnosis of AS. Learning about it can help you to accept it and focus on helping your child.

- Parents sometimes feel guilty, wondering what they did to cause AS or because they did not get help for their child earlier.

- Be sure to find time for yourself each day to help reduce stress, recharge, and have a more positive perspective about your child's needs.

- Spouses may disagree about strategies to help their child or may not have time for themselves because of the amount of time it takes to care for their Aspie. Couples need to work on maintaining communication and continue to connect with one another.

chapter 21

Creating an Asperger-Friendly Home

Creating a semblance of order in your household

The downside of too much structure

Suggestions for setting rules

Setting up rewards and consequences

As parents, we naturally impose structure into our children's lives. Running our households depends on it; we must have some semblance of order to get everyone up and out of the house each morning. And in the evening we must manage dinner, activities, and homework to end the day peacefully before tucking each child into bed at night. Children with Asperger's syndrome (AS) need structure; they need to know what to expect and what their role in the household is. This structure provides a sense of security in an otherwise chaotic world.

Structure, however, must take into account your child's sense of right and wrong and his logical, linear thinking process. He has beliefs about how things should be done and doesn't easily adapt when situations don't mesh with his ideas. Structure, therefore, should include his input. For example, when your child is young, he may want (and need) toys put away in a certain order or placed on the shelf in a certain way. Imposing your views on how the toys should be put away will probably end up in a power struggle. Instead you might insist that toys be off the floor and put away by a certain time each evening but leave how they are put away up to him, integrating his internal sense of order into your decision.

<table>
<tr><td>The Doctor's Take</td><td>We hear all the time about the need for structure in the lives of Aspies. Often it isn't structure but the opposite—variation—that is needed. We have a saying at our clinic—"Life happens!" It is important to teach your child to cope with the unexpected. This isn't easy, but it could be rewarding and important. Plan irregularities in your child's schedule. Practice what to do if something they expect doesn't happen. Anticipate the unexpected and prepare your child to positively approach managing change.</td></tr>
</table>

Parents need to observe their child to find out what will work best. Annie has three children, and her youngest, Tommy, has AS. She has always insisted on a specific schedule after school. When her children arrived home, they had a snack and then did their homework. But Tommy didn't fit into this structure. School, with all the continuous activity, was often overwhelming for him, and he needed more than a short snack break before doing his homework. At first, Annie insisted all three children follow her after-school schedule. The older two had no problem, but Tommy was consistently frustrated and irritated while doing homework; on many days meltdowns occurred, and the entire evening was strained. Annie decided to talk to Tommy about what he thought was best.

Although he couldn't explain that he was overwhelmed and needed extra time, he did say that when he was frustrated at school, he thought about his trains to help calm him down. Annie decided to use this and told Tommy he could come home, have a snack, and play with his trains for one hour before doing his homework. Each day she set a timer for one hour, and it was Tommy's responsibility to stop playing with the trains when the timer went off and start on his homework. Once Annie took Tommy's individual needs into account, homework time and the rest of the evening went much more smoothly.

Using this type of approach helps parents maintain structure but allows for flexibility. This can sometimes create other problems. For example, Annie's other children might resent that Tommy gets to play for an hour before doing homework while they don't have that choice. They may think that Tommy's needs are more important than their own. Finding the right approach, creating structure while taking into account the entire family's needs rather than creating structure around one person's needs, is often a balancing act.

Dinner at 6:30 Sharp

MISC.

Rhonda and her husband, Greg, arrived home from work at 5:30 each day, and dinner was on the table at 6:30. Their son, Andy, completed his homework after school with his babysitter and then watched two videos. When the second video was over, it was dinner time. One evening, Rhonda and Greg had plans to go out. They arrived home early and had dinner ready for Andy at 5:30. Andy refused to eat; the second video was just starting. He couldn't adjust to a change in schedule.

Another question for families is how much structure is too much? There is a danger to making household routines too rigid. One downfall of too much structure is it can increase your child's rigid thinking and reduce his ability to adapt to change. Aspies tend to think in black and white with little use for the gray areas in between, which can lead to problems when schedules must be changed. Creating a routine and structure but introducing small changes allows your child the structure he needs but aids him in developing flexibility.

Setting Ground Rules

Some parents of Aspies find discipline is the least of their problems. Their children have a strong sense of right and wrong and find it hard to break the rules. They only need to explain a rule once, and as long as the rule makes sense, their child will follow it to a tee. Your child may need to see the logic behind the rule, with specific, concrete consequences listed. For example, if you are explaining it is rude to interrupt others, an explanation of "people won't like you" is too abstract. Your child knows there are levels to "not liking" and wonders what this statement means exactly. Instead, say something like, "If you continue to interrupt others when they are talking, your classmates will stop including you in conversations." Start out by acknowledging that everyone makes mistakes, and that they are not a reason to get stressed. How you handle a mistake, learning from it, and avoiding the same one in the future is itself an important life skill.

There will be times your child does something you find inappropriate or unacceptable. At these times, you need to explain what he did that was wrong, why it was wrong, and what he should have done. If your child is in the middle of a meltdown, it is best to wait until later, when the meltdown is over and he is calm. Later, talk about what happened; start by listening. Many times misbehavior is a result of a miscommunication or a misunderstanding; he may have taken something literally that should not have been or been seen as talking back when he was "telling the truth." Lecturing him about the correct behavior won't work until you understand why he did what he did; remember—all behavior is a form of communication. Use the situation as an opportunity to explain the rule that was broken and how rules can have different interpretations in different situations.

Using rewards and consequences as the basis to your household ground rules tends to work best; however, discipline should focus more on rewards for appropriate behaviors than on the consequences for inappropriate behaviors. Think of this as "crowding out" the weeds or inappropriate behaviors by nurturing the flowers or positive behaviors. Recognize and praise good behavior, letting your child know how you expect him to act. Keep in mind that all behavior is communication. Before reacting with a consequence for bad behavior, think about what your Aspie is trying to tell you. Is he overwhelmed? Is he frustrated? Use common sense and don't overreact; make sure the punishment fits the crime.

Following are some ideas to keep in mind when setting up ground rules for your household:

Use a take-away approach rather than a time-out. Using time-outs is sometimes counterproductive. Your child might welcome the chance to retreat to his room, spending time pursuing his passions. Instead, focus consequences on taking away something for a short period of time. You might take away a favorite toy or time spent on the computer. Remember, for this to be effective, you have to tailor it to your child's specific motivators.

Choose your battles. This is especially important with teens. You will sometimes need to allow them to make their own choices and live with the consequences, good and bad. Focus instead on issues that may impact their health or safety.

Avoid using threats. Don't threaten your child with punishment if you are not willing to follow through.

Review rules that aren't working. If you find you are repeating yourself, such as "I told you already to make your bed," you need to review the rule, the consequence, and your behavior to find out why it isn't working. Often, breaking down the task into smaller increments works well.

Institute a tangible consequence for when your child hurts someone. Besides saying he is sorry, give specific steps your child must take to make amends. For example, you might have him do something nice, like write an apology note or share homemade cookies with the other person.

Use rewards that motivate your child. Each child is different—some will respond to staying up late to watch a favorite television show, and teens and older children might respond to monetary or physical type rewards. Many parents will use their child's passion or special interest as a way to reward appropriate behavior.

Be consistent when enforcing rules. Don't ignore the behavior one time and discipline for the behavior the next time. Once you have established a rule, enforce it the very first time it is broken. Avoid changing the rule or the consequences after you have set up a rule, as this is confusing for your child. Carpenters have an old saying: measure twice, cut once. When setting limits for a child, it should be "think twice before speaking, but once you have set a limit, enforce it."

The Doctor's Take

We try to take a positive approach by figuring out what purpose a problem behavior serves and developing an appropriate, alternative behavior to take its place. Then we focus on practicing the replacement behavior. We also stay focused on giving more intense praise and rewards when the child demonstrates the new behavior spontaneously. We also try to reserve punishment for more serious issues, particularly health and safety issues, so that when it is needed, it is more effective and not burned out from overuse.

No matter what discipline methods you use in your house, make sure you and your husband are "on the same page." Spend time when your children are not around to discuss household rules and what rewards and consequences are most appropriate. Be proactive by listing common behaviors and how they should be handled, as well as what your basic household rules are. Write down what you both decide is best so that no matter who is home the same rules are enforced, and the same rewards and consequences are followed. Post your rules in a place everyone can see them; your child will know exactly what is expected and what will happen if he does not follow the rules.

Implementing a Token Economy

Aspies can have a hard time with internal motivation; your child follows rules because the rule makes sense, not because "he did a good job." He may not feel the same pride as others when overcoming a challenging situation. Instead, he is motivated by *instant gratification* or a "what's in it for me" mentality. Token economies focus on rewarding desired behaviors, are easy to set up and maintain, and work well both at home and at school.

> **Definition**
>
> **Instant gratification** refers to a person wanting something immediately. This can sometimes result in poor behavior, grabbing a toy from another child because he wants it, or hitting someone because it felt good in the moment. Young children usually don't understand waiting for something but usually develop this understanding as they mature. Aspies, however, don't always grow out of wanting instant gratification.

Steps for setting up a token economy:

1. Select one behavior you want to improve. It is best to start out working only on one behavior at a time; depending on your child, you can work on two behaviors after he gets used to how a token economy works. More than two behaviors are often too overwhelming.

2. State the desired behavior. Use specific, concrete terms for what behavior you expect. For example, "hand in homework every day" or "get dressed without assistance."

3. Decide what type of tokens you will use. Some examples include poker chips or coins. If you are not using coins, decide on a point value for your tokens. You might decide that each day your child gets dressed without help he gets one point or one token.

4. Choose rewards. Rewards should be based on something that will motivate your child. It can be money, a toy, extra time on the computer, or extra time to pursue their passion. It is more effective to give a menu of rewards, allowing your child to choose what he wants. Place a value on each reward, for example, an extra hour on the computer could be worth 5 points, so if your child gets dressed without assistance every day before school, he will have received 5 tokens, and on the weekend can "purchase" extra time. Make certain that you have several layers, or values, of rewards available so that if he does not have a perfect week and only gets 4 tokens, he still has something for which he can exchange his tokens. Layering the rewards is a step most often skipped or missed and can really make the entire process much more likely to work.

5. Decide how you will monitor your child's progress. Be as specific as possible. What does "getting dressed without assistance" mean? Is your child expected to have all clothes, shoes, and socks on before he comes down for breakfast? If he has the most trouble with shoes, are they not necessary to earn the token? Make sure that your child understands exactly what is expected of him and how both of you will know whether he succeeded. If possible, have your child track his own behaviors.

6. Choose a date to start the program.

Token economies are often extremely effective with Aspies. Your child receives immediate feedback each time you give him a token, but at the same time you're teaching him to wait as he must collect a certain number of tokens before he can "purchase" a reward. Remember, the point of a token economy is to have your child succeed; make sure the goals you set for your child are attainable, and as well as giving a token, praise your child's progress.

Aspie Advice

For an older child, in middle or high school, monetary rewards work well. There is often some gadget he wants to save for, and this gives him the opportunity to learn to budget his money and save for a desired item. If it is a large item, you might want to add in some small rewards along the way to keep up motivation.

Some families add "fines" to a token economy, taking away tokens for undesired behaviors. If you are working on "getting dressed without assistance," your child earns a token each morning he dresses by himself. If you need to step in and help, you take a token away. If you decide to have rewards and fines, wait until after your child has worked with the token economy and has achieved some success before taking away tokens.

Fines have a definite potential downside that you should consider—they can increase the likelihood of a tantrum or aggression in children who are already prone to those behaviors. In cases in which the child is already displaying tantrums or aggression, the token economy is more likely to be an asset if you focus solely on positive rewards and do not include a fine system.

Some additional tips for creating a token economy include:

- For very young children, choose a behavior that occurs several times per day and "catch" him in the desired behavior so he understands how the program works. Because young children have a hard time waiting for rewards, you might want to allow him to cash in his tokens each night and slowly spread it out to every other night, every four days, and finally once a week.

- Remember that it is an "economy" so you can work on both the reward distribution (how much pay is earned for good work) and the costs involved (how many tokens each item costs). As the program continues and desired behaviors become more frequent, the value of the tokens should decrease, as you work on maintaining the behavior over time. Token economies can be very useful in teaching children math and economics skills.

- When you have reached a level where you are satisfied with your child's behavior, you can add a behavior and start the process over.

Essential Takeaways

- Structure is important to an Aspie, but too much structure promotes rigidity.
- Rules should be explained in specific, concrete terms.
- Writing down and posting rules makes sure everyone in the family understands exactly what is expected and what the consequences are for not following the rules.
- Token economies provide instant feedback for good behaviors and help teach delayed gratification.

chapter 22

Siblings

Finding time for all your children

Making chore time family time

Accepting changing emotions in siblings

Helping create lasting sibling relationships

Each child has specific needs; as a parent you work toward making sure your children have all of their needs taken care of, even when that means you must treat them differently. When one of your children has Asperger's syndrome (AS), those differences become more pronounced. Your Aspie may need extra time and attention, leaving your other children feeling as if they aren't as important to you. In this chapter, we talk about the impact of AS on siblings and how you, as a parent, can help siblings adapt to and thrive with a sibling with special needs.

Giving Everyone Time and Attention

Risa looked over at her two children, quietly eating a snack while watching television, and sighed in relief. Jack had come home from school frustrated and angry, and she had spent an hour dealing with him, calming him down before the whole house exploded. Now Jack was in his room, reading one of his favorite books, and she was exhausted. She was thankful that his two older siblings didn't need so much intensive attention and took the initiative to take care of their own needs.

But then Risa felt guilty; didn't they deserve her attention, too? Shouldn't she be there for them when they came home, and listen to what happened at school? Now she felt rushed. It was time to make dinner and get on to homework, but she knew it was also important to take some time to talk to Jenny and Kurt. She didn't want them to feel that they were only important if it was convenient for her. So with a deep breath, she went in, turned off the television, sat down, and gave them both a big hug, saying, "How was your day at school?" Dinner could wait a little while longer.

When you have a child with AS, this scenario might be too familiar. You regret the time you don't spend with your other children, but at the same time you don't know what to do, and your Aspie needs you and frequently needs you "right now." You rely on siblings to take more responsibility for their own care because it gives you time to deal with the immediate needs of their brother or sister. But that approach usually brings guilt and feelings of inadequacy. What kind of a parent are you to ignore some of your children?

It is easy to fall into a pattern of giving your Aspie the attention he needs and then focusing on your other children, with whatever time and energy is left. But this leaves questions in siblings' minds: "Do you love him more than me?" "Am I less important?" Our children want our attention and our love and will adjust their own behavior to get it. They may be well behaved, sometimes too well behaved, trying to live up to our expectations.

Or your child may go the other way, acting out to get your attention. He sees that his brother gets your attention by having a meltdown and decides that is the only time you pay attention to someone. And so he acts out—hitting others, yelling, screaming, and not doing schoolwork. His behavior might be saying, "Remember me? I need you, too."

The following are some ideas to help create a more "family friendly" environment in your home:

When everyone arrives home, whether after school or after work, take 15 minutes to sit together. Don't rush to make dinner or hurry to care for the needs of one particular child. Instead, insist on a few minutes to talk together, letting your children know you are excited to be with them again. Have questions ready for each child, such as "What was your favorite part of today?" or "How did your math test go?" Rotate who you talk to first and give each child a specific time to talk, making sure no one person monopolizes your family time. Your conversations can be continued around the dinner table later.

Make sure each child gets private time with you every day or every week. This may be reading a story together each night at bedtime and then spending a few minutes privately, going out to get ice cream together, or playing a game. No matter how you and your child connect, it is important for each child to have you to himself at some point during the week. Enlist the help of your spouse, letting him be responsible for the other children, sometimes trading places so he can also connect individually with your children.

Aspie Advice	Recognize and praise each child's uniqueness and contributions to the family. Take time each day to appreciate how each person fits into the family and how their talents and skills are important.

Create rules that fit your entire household, and enforce rules for everyone. Make sure you aren't excusing your Aspie's behavior because he can't help it or because he has a disability. Make sure your rules focus on the household, not on individual children.

Encourage all of your children, including any children with AS, to do whatever tasks are possible on their own. If your Aspie has trouble completing certain chores or tasks on his own, adjust the tasks so he can complete tasks on his own and build self-confidence. Set goals to help each child work toward independence and self-reliance.

Before assisting your children, think about whether this task is something they can do themselves. Adjust how you approach tasks to allow your children to complete at least a portion of the task on their own.

Use chores as a way to have family time. Clean the house or do yard work as a family, dividing chores according to each child's ability. Working together to accomplish something will help all your children feel part of the family.

Schedule family outings. This might be a trip to the playground, a museum, or going out to dinner. You may need to take into consideration your Aspie when planning the outings, but be sure to include your other children's interests to let them know you think they are important as well.

Helping Siblings Cope

When children have a sibling with AS, they often grow up more tolerant of differences, but this starts with your attitude. How you treat your Aspie at home is reflected by how your other children treat not only their sibling but others who are considered "different" or have disabilities. Some become "protectors" of their sibling and classmates who have difficulties, befriending the friendless or always volunteering to be partners during group projects.

MISC.	**Eating Lunch Alone**
	Becky's younger brother has AS. She knows how difficult it is for him to make friends and that it hurts him to spend so much time alone. At school, Becky is known for befriending the friendless. In the cafeteria, whenever she sees someone sitting alone, Becky invites him or her to sit at her lunch table. Becky's friends don't understand, sometimes resenting the intrusion, but they have come to accept that is just the way Becky is.

Your other children may resent the differences, feeling they have to give up too much in order to accommodate their sibling's needs. Your choices of restaurants or vacations may revolve around your Aspie, rather than taking into consideration everyone's interests or likes. They may feel you are more lenient on their sibling and too harsh on them. They may think they always have to be the accommodating or understanding one and not understand why the Aspie can't make compromises as well.

Aspies have often been described as "odd" or "quirky," and your non-Aspie children, especially when they reach the preteen and teen years, want to fit in, without drawing too much attention to their differences. They may be faced with remarks, insults, or teasing from classmates because their sibling is strange or acts weird. Siblings might feel they are put on the spot, having to defend their sibling from teasing but at the same time being embarrassed by his actions. This can create complex and sometimes conflicting emotional states.

Changing Roles

MISC.

Cassie's role as big sister continuously changed. One day, Cassie was angry. Todd was acting up. She wanted to tell their mom about getting a part in the school play, but Todd was having a bad day and all her mom did was pay attention to him. "He ruins everything," Cassie thought. But the next day when one of the older kids teased Todd, Cassie was right by his side, holding his hand, being the protective, caring big sister.

Emotions can run high for everyone in the family, and communication is often the most important tool for effective coping. Here are a few key things to consider for your family.

As parents, it is always important to keep up communication between you and your children, and this is even more important when one of your children has AS. Siblings need to be able to talk about their feelings; allow them to express their frustration, anger, or concern for and about their brother or sister. You should keep in mind that feelings can change from day to day; one day the sibling may be the protector, another day she is angry that the Aspie embarrassed her in front of her friends. When you, as parents, know and accept that feelings can and will change from day to day, or even moment to moment, and let your child know you love her no matter what, it goes a long way toward validating her feelings.

It is helpful to set clear expectations for all your children. Often, siblings don't understand what their brother or sister can do and can't do and will lower expectations for the Aspie, helping with homework, doing chores, or watching over him at school. While some siblings might think parents are too lenient, others will believe parents expect too much of the Aspie and try to compensate by helping, setting aside their needs to do so. You can help by setting realistic goals for each child based on his abilities and celebrating each child's successes. Explain to siblings that it is important to allow the Aspie to try and to reach his own goals and reach for independence.

Make sure siblings have someone to talk to. Some AS groups and programs have separate groups for siblings, giving them a chance to share stories and support one another. Siblings may not have anyone in their lives who understands. Most of their friends have no concept of how their daily lives have ups and downs based on their sibling with AS's moods or how difficult it can be at times to communicate with their sibling. They, just like you, need others in their lives who let them know they are not alone.

The most important way to help siblings cope is by giving them information about AS. Let them know what it is, how it impacts their sibling's life, what treatments are, and why they are needed. Remember that as the siblings grow and mature, you will need to update the information. Understanding what is going on and why can help them better focus on positive ways to help the Aspie.

Building Sibling Relationships

Aspies often have few, if any, relationships outside the family. Their siblings are their first and, in many cases, their most important relationships. Their siblings will be in their lives longer than anyone else, and their relationships with siblings will provide the Aspie with an enormous amount of information on how to relate to others.

> **Aspie Advice**
>
> Non-Aspie siblings may be frustrated with the inability to emotionally connect with their sibling. They may feel the Aspie is selfish and doesn't ever care about anyone else's feelings. Help foster empathy by helping your Aspie show appreciation and caring. Have him help bake his sister's favorite cookies to congratulate her for a job well done or shop for a gift for her birthday.

Some siblings may resent not having a "normal" relationship with the Aspie. Their friends may be able to joke and tease their siblings, but your Aspie frequently doesn't get the jokes and efforts to tease go flat or end up with the Aspie being angry. Just as you set up play dates and intervene to help your young Aspie learn to get along with other children his age, you may need to do so with your own children. Spending time playing and doing activities as a family helps all of your children be more sensitive to each other's needs and find ways to communicate with one another.

Most siblings get along sometimes and argue at other times; when you have both Aspies and neurotypical children, sibling relationships aren't any different. One minute they will get along, and the next they aren't speaking to one another. As parents, it is hard to watch siblings fight or argue, but remember that sibling relationships are like any other, there are positives and negatives, but in the end, the positives normally outweigh the negatives.

Essential Takeaways

- Siblings may resent the amount of time you must devote to the Aspie; it is important for parents to give each child attention.
- Every child should be appreciated for their uniqueness and the gifts they bring to the family.
- Allow siblings to voice their frustrations about living with a sibling with AS as well as their concern for him.
- Siblings can be one of the most important relationships in your Aspie's life, and this relationship is often the foundation for relationships with peers.

chapter 23

Attending Events

Anticipating problems when away from the house

Staying on schedule

Adjusting expectations

To tell or not to tell: revealing AS to others

Going out to dinner, taking the family for ice cream, and attending family parties are always an adventure, as any parent of a child with Asperger's syndrome (AS) will attest to. Worry about meltdowns or aggressive behavior settles in the back of your mind and remains there. In this chapter, we talk about steps you can take to help your family get through social outings as well as how to handle comments made by well-meaning or misinformed friends and relatives.

Preparing Your Child

The key to making it through any social outing, whether it is a quiet outing with just your immediate family, or a large party filled with relatives, is preparation. Your Aspie needs routine, structure, and predictability, and the more you provide these things, the better the outing will go. This isn't to say that when you prepare your day will go smoothly, but it certainly helps improve the possibility.

Understanding Trouble Spots

Aspies are easily overwhelmed in noisy, crowded environments. Knowing this, and being ready for the unexpected, helps your child better manage high-stimulus events. Before heading out the door, take time to list areas that are potential problems for your child and come up with possible solutions. For example:

Try to divert the overly affectionate. When attending family events, do relatives consistently try to hug and kiss your child, making him uncomfortable? Briefly explain to relatives that he does not like to be hugged but will be glad to shake hands. Prepare him by practicing having him hold his hand out for a handshake rather than a hug.

> **The Doctor's Take**
>
> Sensory issues won't disappear by ignoring whatever is causing the problem. Your child can't ignore the bright lights or tune out the overwhelming noises. As a parent, you can help to filter out some of the bothersome stimulus if you understand what causes him the most difficulty. For example, if he is sensitive to noise, have him keep an iPod with him so he can listen to calming music through headphones and ignore the loud noises around him.

Locate a quiet space. When visiting relatives, is there a private room or area your child can retreat to for quiet time? Contact relatives beforehand and ask whether there is a den or bedroom that can be designated as a quiet area for your child. If going to the mall, look for an out-of-the-way spot you can go to if your child becomes stressed or plan on retreating to your car for a few minutes.

Bring along some favorite items. Will the event be noisy or crowded, leading to possible sensory overload? Prepare by letting your child choose a few toys related to his passion so he can retreat by himself and get away from the noise.

Time your shopping trips around your child's needs. If you are going shopping, especially during the holidays, do the noise, the crowds, and the hustle and bustle, lead to feelings of being overwhelmed? Talk to your child beforehand and schedule shopping trips during off-peak hours or if that is not possible, consider using a babysitter and shopping alone.

Make sure there are food choices your child likes. Does a restaurant offer food choices your child will eat? Aspies often eat only a limited number of foods; check online to find out if there is something your child will like. If not, consider a different restaurant, or, if that is not possible, pack some snacks for him. This applies to visiting relatives' homes as well. If you aren't sure whether he will eat the food at your relative's home, bring along food for him so you aren't dealing with a hungry, overwhelmed child.

Take steps to ensure your child is included in activities. When attending family functions, are there cousins or other children that tease or exclude your child? Family events should be a safe and secure place where your child feels accepted for who he is. If he doesn't get along with relatives, find an older relative or sibling who can spend time with your child and be in charge of making sure he is included in games and activities.

Thinking about possible problems and solutions before you leave your house helps the entire family enjoy the outing and relieves the stress for your Aspie, you, and your spouse.

Creating a Schedule

We all believe spontaneity adds spice to life, but in the world of Aspies, spontaneity adds feelings of being overwhelmed and can lead to inappropriate or embarrassing behaviors. Creating a schedule does not mean you have to list what is going to happen every minute of the day. However, your Aspie does need to know what to expect and when to expect it.

A couple examples of schedules for family outings:

> *Going out to dinner*
>
> 5:00: Leaving
>
> 5:15: Arrive at restaurant
>
> We will wait to be seated and then look over the menu and order our food
>
> 6:30: We should be done eating and heading home

Based on your individual child, you can include more detail, or you can give an overview of what is going to happen, explaining to your child that you can't predict exactly what time you will be seated or what time you will be done. It might help for you to check the restaurant's website and choose meals before you arrive.

When going out to dinner, it is sometimes helpful to have a favorite or regular restaurant. Your Aspie will feel more comfortable in a familiar place. You can ask the manager if you can take a menu home, allowing your children to make their selections before you leave the house, avoiding indecision or long discussions about choices while sitting at the restaurant.

Attending a family party

2:00: Leaving

2:30: We should arrive at Aunt Mary's house

2:30 until 4:00: "Social" time before dinner; spend time in playroom with cousins

4:00: Dinner

5:00: "Social" time while adults clean up after dinner and say their good-byes

6:00: Leaving for home

By providing your child with a schedule, letting him know when you are leaving, when you are expected to arrive, and what he will be doing during the visit, he can better prepare.

Going Over the Rules

For the most part, rules are rules; the expectations for your child's behavior in your house are the same as those when he is in a friend's or relative's house. Even so, there are often times when adjustments need to be made to behavior. For example, does your child need to ask before getting up from the table or sit quietly while everyone else finishes their meal? You need to be specific about your expectations, letting your child know rewards and consequences for appropriate and inappropriate behaviors.

Aunt Mary's House

misc.

Anna and her family were heading to Aunt Mary's house for a visit. When company was over or at snack time, Anna usually let the children take their plates and eat in the family room, but she knew this wasn't allowed at Aunt Mary's house. Before leaving her house, she explained the different set of rules, stating that everyone must sit at the kitchen table when eating anything—meals and snacks. Sometimes, she explained, there are different rules at different houses.

Whether you are visiting relatives for an afternoon or for the weekend, eating out, or going shopping, sit down and explain the rules in advance. Make sure your child knows exactly what is expected of him. Go through the event from beginning to end; for example, start from the time you leave the house and include the following:

- Where you are going

- What time you expect to arrive

- How long you will be staying

- A schedule about what is going on

- Any special instructions, such as greeting relatives, where he can go when he needs quiet time, and specific rules for the house you are visiting

Keep your perspective on the event realistic. If you want perfection, you will probably be disappointed. Instead, enjoy what you are doing and accept that your "normal" may not always be the same as other people's "normal." Focus on the positives and put aside the belief that you and your family must live up to other people's expectations.

Talking About Asperger's Syndrome

Whether or not you choose to tell friends and relatives that your child has AS is a personal decision. Talk to your spouse and find out whether or not he is comfortable disclosing your child's diagnosis; if your child is old enough, include him in the discussion. What does he feel comfortable sharing? Would explaining AS make him uncomfortable? Decide, as a family, how much information, if any, you want to share with others and with whom you want to share this information.

> **Aspie Advice**
>
> When deciding who to disclose your child's diagnosis to, think about how much contact this person will have with him. You may want to tell close family members and friends who have regular contact with him, but relatives who are seen only once or twice a year probably don't need to know.

There may be certain behaviors, such as repetitive behaviors or meltdowns, that are obvious to others, and you feel you need to explain. Because AS is a spectrum disorder, your child may not have any symptoms that are obvious to others, and in these cases many families choose not to say anything.

What to Say

If you decide to discuss your child's diagnosis, plan what you want to say ahead of time. Although each situation is different, the following are some suggestions on explaining AS:

Explain that your child has difficulty communicating his needs. You may want to compare it to being in another country and not being able to speak the language. You know what you want but can't make others understand. You can hear other people talking, but can't make sense of what they are saying. Explain that using simple sentences, free of figures of speech and idioms, is best when talking to your child.

Discuss some of the main symptoms that they may see. For instance, lack of eye contact, resisting changes, difficulty transitioning from one activity to another, sensory sensitivities, and not being able to show or explain emotion. Let friends and relatives know that these behaviors are not him being rude.

> **Misc.**
>
> **Reacting to Disbelief**
>
> Sasha's son, age 13, was recently diagnosed with AS. When Sasha told her sister about the diagnosis, the response was, "I don't think he has autism; he talks too much. You should get a second opinion." Sasha was ready for her sister's disbelief and took out a list of books and reputable websites. She explained that she agreed with the diagnosis. Instead of arguing, Sasha asked her sister to read more about AS and then come back with questions. As far as Sasha was concerned, the discussion was over.

When your child behaves inappropriately, let friends and relatives know that he is not trying to be contrary. Explain this behavior usually occurs because there is something he doesn't understand. Taking the time to view the situation from his perspective and explaining what is going on works better than punishing him for his behaviors.

Remind friends and relatives that AS is not an illness or a disease, but rather it is a different way of being. Explain that your son processes information differently but does not have "mental illness" or a behavioral disorder.

Handling Negative Comments

No matter how much you try to explain AS in a calm and informative way, frequently at least one person makes negative comments about your child's behavior or thinks you are using the diagnosis as an excuse to accept poor behavior. In other words, she believes your parenting has caused your child's AS. Before getting angry, decide whether this person is worth your anger or your time. If she is a relative you see once a year, do you want to ruin your time trying to get her to understand?

You may hear a comment such as, "My neighbor has a child with AS, and he doesn't act like that. He is always very quiet …" You might want to explain that AS is a spectrum disorder, and everyone with AS is different, just like every child is different. Some may be quiet; some may not.

Another frustrating remark parents hear is, "He just needs some discipline." Although comments such as these are hurtful, it is important to remember that those making comments do not live in your home. They are basing their opinion on their own experiences. Be confident in your abilities as a parent. Know that you have done your research, you know your child, and you know what is best for him. If you do choose to respond, take care of your child first, and show through your actions that your child is more important than their opinion in your life.

For some parents, it is easier to simply walk away from negative comments. You know your son, you know what causes his behaviors, and you know what is best. If listening to those who don't understand and believe inaccurate information makes you upset, it may be best to focus your energies on taking care of your family and leave the situation.

Essential Takeaways

- Thinking about potential problems and coming up with solutions before going out with your child can make outings more peaceful.

- Give your child a schedule of your outing, including when you are leaving, how long you will be there, and what time you expect to be home.

- Be clear on what your expectations are before you leave for a family event or a shopping trip.

- If your child is old enough, include him in discussions as to whether to disclose his AS diagnosis.

Appendix A

Glossary

accommodations   Changes instituted in school or in the workplace to allow for challenges based on a disability.

anxiety disorders   A disorder characterized by extreme worry and nervousness.

Applied Behavior Analysis (ABA)   Method used to reduce or minimize inappropriate behaviors or to build on daily living skills and communication skills. It uses the concept of positive reinforcement for desired behaviors and no reaction for undesired behaviors.

Asperger's syndrome   A neurological disorder characterized by an unusual and intense preoccupation with a subject, impaired social and communication skills, and repetitive behaviors.

Aspie   A term commonly used to refer to an individual with Asperger's disorder.

assistive technology   Any item, product, or piece of equipment that is used to help someone with a disability.

Attention Deficit Hyperactivity Disorder (ADHD) A neurobiological disorder characterized by hyperactivity, inattention, and impulsiveness.

autism   A developmental disorder that appears within the first three years of life and affects social and communication skills.

autism spectrum disorder   A group of developmental disorders also known as pervasive developmental disorders (PDD). Besides Asperger's syndrome, this group includes autistic disorder, pervasive development disorder—not otherwise specified, Rett syndrome, and childhood disintegrative disorder.

behavior analysis   An approach that observes and investigates behaviors and then applies that information to an individual to help improve behavior.

cognitive behavioral therapy (CBT)   Therapy to change the way a person thinks and reacts to stimuli. It can include exposure or desensitization exercises.

cognitive skills   The ability to learn and use or thoughts, experiences, and senses to obtain and understand information.

depression   A mental illness characterized by feelings of sadness, discouragement, or hopelessness that lasts for weeks or months.

Diagnostic and Statistical Manual **(DSM)**   The standard diagnostic reference for mental illnesses, published by the American Psychiatric Association.

disorder of written expression   A learning disability characterized by poor writing skills, such as illegible handwriting and frequent errors in spelling and punctuation.

Early Intervention (EI)   A support system for young children, up to age 3, with developmental disabilities or delays including evaluation and individual services, such as speech, occupational, or physical therapy.

evidence-based treatments   Treatments that have been proven to work through rigorous research, such as random, double-blind studies or the collection and interpretation of data from patients, doctors, and research.

giftedness   A significantly higher than average intellectual ability.

high-functioning autism   A term used to describe individuals with autism and language delays who have developed the ability to speak in complex sentences.

hypersensitivities   *See* sensory sensitivities.

hypotonia   A generalized muscle weakness that can affect posture, movement, strength, and coordination.

idiom   An expression of speech in which the meaning cannot be derived by using context clues, and is often used by a particular group of people.

Individualized Educational Plan (IEP)   A legally binding document that lists and explains what special education services a child will receive.

instant gratification   Wanting something immediately, sometimes resulting in poor behavior.

life coach   A person who works with individuals based on specific needs, such as organization, social skills, or conflict resolution.

meltdowns   Similar to a severe or extreme temper tantrum but usually caused by overstimulation or sensory overload.

multisensory   Approaches that incorporate two or more of the senses during the learning process.

neurotypical   A term used to describe people without autism or Asperger's syndrome.

nonverbal learning disorder (NVLD)   A learning disability characterized by deficits in perception, coordination, socialization, nonverbal problem solving, an understanding of humor or sarcasm, and a highly developed rote memory.

obsession   A fixation on an idea, object, or person. Thoughts and ideas about the obsession intrude in a person's thoughts and interfere with normal functioning for that person.

obsessive compulsive disorder (OCD)   A type of anxiety disorder characterized by obsessive, intrusive thoughts and compulsions, tasks, or rituals, which are done over and over in an effort to reduce or stop the obsessions.

occupational therapy   A type of treatment that works with people in carrying out daily activities.

passions   A term used to describe the intense, focused special interests of individuals on the autism spectrum.

perfectionism   A belief that it is unacceptable to make any mistakes or errors while performing an activity.

pervasive development disorder   A developmental disability characterized by delays in basic functioning, including socialization and communication.

physical therapy   A type of treatment that focuses on body movement and provides customized treatments to help individuals perform physical tasks and improve movement.

pragmatics   Studying and using language in a social context.

prosody   The pitch, rhythm, stress, and melody of speech.

rating scale   A diagnostic tool requiring the person completing it to rate behaviors or abilities from low to high.

repetitive behaviors   Physical or verbal behaviors that are continually repeated, such as repeating a phrase over and over or waving hands.

rituals   Specific behaviors that are repeated in a certain way in order to provide a sense of security, such as lining up toys in a certain way or going through a set of behaviors before bed each night.

ruminate   To think deeply about a subject, to turn it over and over in the mind beyond that which is typical under similar circumstances.

schizophrenia   A mental disorder characterized by the inability to know the difference between real and unreal experiences.

Section 504   A civil rights law that protects a child from being discriminated against in the school setting.

sensory sensitivities   Being either over- or underresponsive to sensory input; for example, sensitivity to touch is common in children with AS.

significant impairment   The level of symptoms interferes with your child's ability to complete or participate in normal daily activities compared to other children their age.

social stories   Developed by Carol Gray, a tool used to describe social situations to help children understand appropriate responses.

special interest   An intense focused interest in a narrow topic.

spectrum disorder   A disorder that includes symptoms which range from mild to severe.

temper tantrum   An expression of anger, often accompanied by physical and verbal outbursts.

token economy   A positive discipline method that allows a child to earn rewards for appropriate and desired behaviors.

Tourette's syndrome   A neuropsychiatric disorder characterized by repetitive and involuntary movements and vocal behaviors called tics.

visual representation system   Objects, photographs, drawings, or written words to enhance the spoken word.

Resources

National Organizations

American Aspergers Association
1301 Seminole Boulevard, B-112
Largo, FL 33770
717-518-7294
www.americanaspergers.org

Asperger Syndrome Coalition of the U.S.
2020 Pennsylvania Avenue NW
PO Box 771
Washington, DC 20006
866-427-7747
www.asperger.org

Autism Society of America
4340 East-West Highway, Suite 350
Bethesda, MD 20814
800-328-8476
www.autism-society.org

Autism Speaks
1 East 33rd Street, 4th Floor
New York, NY 10016
212-252-8584
www.autismspeaks.org

National Autism Center
41 Pacella Park Drive
Randolph, MA 02368
877-313-3833
www.nationalautismcenter.org

Special Needs Alliance
6342 East Brian Kent Drive
Tucson, AZ 85710
877-572-8472
www.specialneedsalliance.com

U.S. Autism & Asperger Association
PO Box 532
Draper, UT 84020-0532
801-816-1234
www.usautism.org

Advocacy Resources and Legal Information

GRASP—The Global and Regional Asperger Syndrome Partnership
666 Broadway, Suite 825
New York, NY 10012
888-474-7277
www.grasp.org

Support Groups

Asperger's Syndrome Meetup Groups
www.aspergers.meetup.com

Listing of Asperger's Support Groups Around the U.S.
www.parentingaspergerscommunity.com/public/department65.cfm

Magazines and Publications

Autism Asperger's Digest
PO Box 2257
Burlington, NC 27216
336-222-0442
www.autismdigest.com

Books to Share with Your Children

Hoopmann, Kathy. *All Cats Have Asperger Syndrome*. London: Jessica Kingsley Publishers, 2006.

Jackson, Luke. *Freaks, Geeks & Asperger Syndrome: A Guide to Adolescence*. London: Jessica Kingsley Publishers, 2002.

Larson, Elaine Marie. *I Am Utterly Unique: Celebrating the Strengths of Children with Asperger Syndrome and High Functioning Autism*. Overland Park: Autism Asperger Publishing Company, 2006.

Patrick, Nancy J. *Social Skills for Teenagers and Adults with Asperger Syndrome*. London: Jessica Kingsley Publishers, 2008.

Books for Parents

Attwood, Tony. *The Complete Guide to Asperger's Syndrome*. London: Jessica Kingsley Publishers, 2008.

Bolick, Teresa. *Asperger Syndrome and Adolescence: Helping Preteens & Teens Get Ready for the Real World*. Minneapolis: Fair Winds Press, 2004.

Mertz, Christine, and Tony Attwood. *Help for the Child with Asperger's Syndrome: A Parent's Guide to Negotiating the Social Service Maze*. London: Jessica Kingsley Publishers, 2004.

Stillman, William. *The Everything Parent's Guide to Children with Asperger's Syndrome*. Avon: Adams Press, 2010.

Zysk, Veronica, and Temple Grandin. *1001 Great Ideas for Teaching and Raising Children with Autism or Asperger's*. Arlington: Future Horizons, 2010.

Websites and Online Resources

Asperger's Association of New England
www.aane.org

Asperger's Syndrome List Subscriber Support
www.asperger.icors.org

Autism Information Center: U.S. Center for Disease Control
www.cdc.gov/ncbddd/autism/index.html

HealthCentral—Autism and Asperger Center
www.healthcentral.com/autism/autism-aspergers-center/

OASIS@MAAP
www.aspergersyndrome.org

Parenting Asperger's Community
www.parentingaspergerscommunity.com

Reinforcement Unlimited Article Index
www.behavior-consultant.com/discussion.htm

Wrong Planet
www.WrongPlanet.net

Your Little Professor
www.yourlittleprofessor.com

References

"About SPD." 16 July (modified 2011). Sensory Processing Disorder Foundation, http://www.spdfoundation. net/about-sensory-processing-disorder.html.

Allman, Toney. *Asperger's Syndrome.* Farmington Hills: Lucent Books, 2009.

Anestis, Michael D. "The Fate of Asperger's Syndrome in DSM-V." 10 Nov 2009. Psychotherapy Brown Bag, http://www.psychotherapybrownbag.com/ psychotherapy_brown_bag_a/2009/11/the-fate-of-aspergers-syndrome-in-dsmv-a-followup-to-last-weeks-article.html.

"Asperger Syndrome." National Alliance on Mental Illness, http://www.nami.org/Content/ ContentGroups/Helpline1/Asperger_Syndrome. htm.

"Asperger Syndrome Fact Sheet." January 2005. National Institute of Neurological Disorders and Stroke, http://www.ninds.nih.gov/disorders/asperger/ detail_asperger.htm.

Attwood, Tony. *The Complete Guide to Asperger's Syndrome.* London: Jessica Kingsley Publishers, 2007.

———. "The Pattern of Abilities and Development of Girls with Asperger's Syndrome." 1999. TonyAtwood.com.au, http://www.tonyattwood. com.au/index.php?Itemid=181&catid=45: archived-resource-papers&id=80:the-pattern-of-abilities-and-development-of-girls-with-aspergers-syndrome&option=com_ content&view=article.

Attwood, Tony, and Lorna Wing. *Asperger's Syndrome: A Guide for Parents and Professionals.* London: Jessica Kingsley Publishing, 1998.

"Autism Spectrum Disorder." 2011. University of Illinois at Chicago, http://ccm.psych.uic.edu/PatientInfo/AutismSpectrumDisorder.aspx.

Bolick, Teresa. *Asperger Syndrome and Adolescence: Helping Preteens & Teens Get Ready for the Real World.* Minneapolis: Fair Winds, 2004.

"Boy with Autism Dies After Chelation Therapy." 25 Aug 2005. MSNBC.com, www.msnbc.msn.com/id/9074208/ns/health-mental_health/t/boy-autism-dies-after-chelation-therapy/#.TksMVmG69C0.

Buckmann, Steve, and Cathy Pratt. "Supporting Students with Asperger's Syndrome Who Present Behavioral Challenges." 1999. Indiana University, http://www.iidc.indiana.edu/?pageId=467.

"Bullying (and Asperger Syndrome)." Your Little Professor, http://www.yourlittleprofessor.com/bullying.html.

Burns, Diane Drake. *Autism, Aspergers, ADHD, ADD: A Parent's Roadmap to Understanding and Support.* Arlington: Future Horizons, 2005.

"But I Can't Live Without It! Managing the Fixations of Children with Asperger's Syndrome." Your Little Professor, http://www.yourlittleprofessor.com/fixations.html.

Clark, Julie. *Asperger's in Pink.* Arlington: Future Horizons, 2010.

Cohen, Jeffrey. *The Asperger Parent.* Shawnee Mission: Autism Asperger Publishing Company, 2002.

Deal vs. Hamilton County School Board. No. 03-5396. U.S. Court of Appeals for the Sixth Circuit. 16 Dec 2004.

"Definition: Idiom." Merriam-Webster.com, http://www.merriam-webster.com/dictionary/idiom.

"Definition: Meltdown." Merriam-Webster.com, http://www.merriam-webster.com/dictionary/meltdown?show=0&t=1311637028.

"Definition: Tantrum." Merriam-Webster.com, http://www.merriam-webster.com/dictionary/tantrum.

Delano, M. E. "Improving Written Language Performance of Adolescents with Asperger Syndrome." *Journal of Applied Behavior Analysis* (2007): 345–351.

Diagnostic and Statistical Manual of Mental Disorders DSM-IV-TR, Fourth Edition (Text Revision). American Psychiatric Association, 2000.

"Do Obsessive Compulsive Disorder (OCD) and Asperger's disorder (AS) co-exist?" 14 Apr 2010. Bio Behavioral Institute, http://www.biobehavioralinstitute.com/viewarticle.php?id=38.

Evans, David W., Kristin Canavera, F. Lee Kleinpeter, Elise Maccubbin, and Ken Taga. "The Fears, Phobias and Anxieties of Children with Autism Spectrum Disorders and Down Syndrome: Comparisons with Developmentally and Chronologically Age Matched Children." *Child Psychiatry and Human Development* (2005): 3–26.

Foden, Teresa, and Connie Anderson. "Bullying and ASD." 25 Aug 2010. Kennedy Krieger Institute, http://www.iancommunity.org/cs/articles/bullying.

Gaus, V. L. *Cognitive-Behavioral Therapy for Adult Asperger Syndrome.* New York: Guilford Press, n.d.

"General Developmental Sequence Toddler through Preschool." Child Development Institute, http://www.childdevelopmentinfo.com/development/devsequence.shtml.

Gernsbacher, Morton Ann. *Toward a Behavior of Reciprocity.* Madison: University of Wisconsin, 2006.

Hoffman, Charles D., Dwight P. Sweeney, James E. Gilliam, Daniel D. Apodaca, Muriel C. Lopez-Wagner, and Melissa M. Castillo. "Sleep Problems and Symptomology in Children with Autism." *Focus on Autism and Other Developmental Disabilities* (2005): 194–201.

"Infant's Movements Can Signal a Form of Autism, UF Study Shows." 26 July 2004. University of Florida News, http://news.ufl.edu/2004/07/26/autismmove/.

Interlandi, Jeneen. "More Than Just 'Quirky.'" *Newsweek Magazine.* 14 Nov 2008.

Knott, Catherine. "Creating a Ring of Courage: Help for the Bullied Child." Learning Disabilities, http://www.learningdisabilitiesinfo. com/bullied-children.html.

Liss, M., J. Mailloux, and M. J. Erchull. "The relationship between sensory processing sensitivity, alexithymia, autism, depression, and anxiety." *Personality and Individual Differences* (2008): 255–259.

Lovendahl, Crisler. "Floortime." Polyxo.com, http://www.polyxo.com/ floortime/buildingplaypartnerships.html#3.4.

McNair, Trisha. "Autism and Asperger Syndrome." BBC Health, http:// www.bbc.co.uk/health/physical_health/conditions/autism1.shtml.

Mertz, Christine, and Tony Attwood. *Help for the Child with Asperger's Syndrome: A Parent's Guide to Negotiating the Social Service Maze.* London: Jessica Kingsley Publishing, 2004.

Myles, B., K. Cook, N. Miller, L. Rinner, and L. Robbins. *Asperger Syndrome and Sensory Issues: Practical Solutions for Making Sense of the World.* Shawnee Mission: Autism Asperger Publishing, 2000.

Myles, B. S., A. Huggins, M. Rome-Lake, T. Hagiwara, G. P. Barnhill, and D. E. Griswold. "Written profiles of children and youth with Asperger syndrome: From research to practice." *Education and Training in Developmental Disabilities* (2003): 362–369.

"NCAHF Policy Statement on Chelation Therapy." 2002. National Council Against Health Fraud, http://www.ncahf.org/policy/chelation.html.

Notbohm, Ellen, and Veronica Zysk. *1001 Great Ideas for Teaching & Raising Children with Autism or Asperger's.* Arlington: Future Horizons, 2010.

Olweus, D. *Bullying at School: What We Know and What We Can Do.* Oxford: Blackwells, 1993.

Olweus, D., and S. Limber. *Blueprints for Violence Prevention: Bullying Prevention Program.* Boulder: Institute of Behavioral Science, 1999.

Olweus Core Program Against Bullying and Antisocial Behavior: A Teacher's Handbook. Bergen: Research Center for Health Promotion, 2001.

Paddock, Catharine. "Early Intervention Very Effective For Toddlers With Autism, Small Study." 30 Nov 2009. Medical News Today, http://www.medicalnewstoday.com/articles/172495.php.

Patrick, Nancy J. *Social Skills for Teenagers and Adults with Asperger Syndrome.* London: Jessica Kingsley Publishers, 2008.

Pellicano, E., M. Mayberry, K. Durkin, and A. Malcy. "Multiple cognitive capabilities/deficits in children with an autism spectrum disorder: 'weak' central coherence and its relationship to theory of mind and executive control." *Developmental Psycopatholgy* (2006): 77–98.

"Pervasive Developmental Disorders." *Diagnostic and Statistical Manual of Mental Disorders, 4th Edition.* Washington, D.C.: American Psychiatric Association, 2000.

"Play Skills-Based Interventions." *Texas Autism Resource Guide for Effective Teaching.* Austin: Texas Statewide Leadership for Autism, 2009.

"Proposed Changes: Autism Spectrum Disorder." 2011. American Psychiatric Association DSM-5 Development, http://www.dsm5.org/ProposedRevision/Pages/proposedrevision.aspx?rid=94#.

Romanowski Bashe, Patricia, and Barbara L. Kirby. *The Oasis Guide to Asperger Syndrome.* New York: Crown Archetype, 2005.

Santomauro, Josie. *Mothering Your Special Child.* London: Jessica Kingsley Publishers, 2009.

Silverman, Stephan M., and Rich Weinfeld. *School Success for Kids With Asperger's Syndrome: A Practical Guide for Parents and Teachers.* Austin: Prufrock Press, Inc., 2007.

Simmons Sicoli, Karen, and Mark Victor Hansen. "Autism and Asperger's Syndrome: Early Warning Signs." Autism Today, http://www.autismtoday.com/articles/wyman.PDF.

Stephens, Laurie. "Understanding Asperger's Disorder in Young Children." 2007. The Help Group, http://www.thehelpgroup.org/pdf/Stephens.pdf.

Stillman, William. *The Everything Parent's Guide to Children with Asperger's Syndrome.* Avon: Adams Media, 2005.

———. *When Your Child Has Asperger's Syndrome.* Avon: Adams Media, 2008.

"Tourette Syndrome Fact Sheet." 15 June (updated 2011). National Institute of Neurological Disorders and Stroke, http://www.ninds.nih.gov/disorders/tourette/detail_tourette.htm.

Wallis, Claudia. "A Powerful Identity, a Vanishing Diagnosis." 2 Nov 2009. The New York Times, http://www.nytimes.com/2009/11/03/health/03asperger.html?pagewanted=1&ref=health.

Welton, Jude. *Can I Tell You About Asperger Syndrome?* London: Jessica Kingsley Publishers, 2004.

"What is Occupational Therapy?" World Federation of Occupational Therapists, http://www.wfot.org/AboutUs/AboutOccupationalTherapy/WhatisOccupationalTherapy.aspx.

Wing, Lorna. "Asperger Syndrome: A Clinical Account." 4 May (updated 2011). Cambridge University Press, http://www.mugsy.org/wing2.htm.

Winter-Messiers, Mary Ann, and Cynthia M. Herr. "Dinosaurs 24/7: Understanding The Special Interests of Children with Asperger's Syndrome." 2 April 2007. Kennedy Krieger Institute, http://www.iancommunity.org/cs/about_asds/the_special_interests_of_children_with_aspergers.

Zysk, Veronica, and Temple Grandin. *1001 Great Ideas for Parenting and Raising Children with Autism or Asperger's.* Arlington: Future Horizons, 2010.

Index

E

R

T